Taste Radiant Living

Taste Radiant Living

7 Simple and Delicious Secrets to Eating and Well-being

Alisha Chasey, MS, RD, CNS
Founder of Innocent Indulgence®

XULON PRESS

Xulon Press
2301 Lucien Way #415
Maitland, FL 32751
407.339.4217
www.xulonpress.com

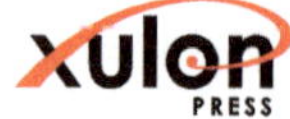

Printed in the United States of America.
Edited by Xulon Press.

ISBN: 9781545616574

Disclaimer

This book contains the opinions and ideas of its author. It is solely for informational and educational purposes and should not be regarded as a substitute for professional medical treatment. Since the nature of your body's health condition is complex and one-of-a kind, it is recommended that you consult with a health professional before you begin any new exercise, nutrition, or supplementation program, or if you have any questions about your health. Neither the author nor the publisher shall be liable or responsible for any reaction, loss or damage, or for any adverse reaction(s) to the consumption of food or products allegedly arising from any information or suggestions in this book. Statements and/or claims in this book about consumable products or food have not been evaluated by the FDA. While the author has made every effort to provide accurate figures and Internet address information at the time of publication, neither the author nor publisher assume any responsibility for errors or changes that occur after publication.

The author and publisher are not responsible for your specific health concerns that may require medical supervision. Individual results may vary. Results or weight loss cannot be guaranteed simply from reading this publication, as they are also dependent on your uniqueness and how you apply the secrets discovered in the pages to follow.

Table of Contents

1. From Cookie Dough to Greens: A Nutritionist's Story (How to Get Started) 1

2. "Healthy" Gets a Makeover: How to Get Motivated 7

Forget the Die-t—Start the Lifestyle!

3. How (and What to Eat) to Make Healthy Delicious . . . 24

Set the Foundation

Make It Colorful

Build Strength and Structure

Spice It Up

4. How to Make Healthy Start with Dessert 47

Naturally Sweet and Sugar-less

5. How to Make Healthy Daily 59

What to Eat

What to Drink

6. How to Make Healthy Doable 87

Making It Happen

Fitting It into Your Wallet and Calendar

Meal and Snack Starters

Shopping Guide

Label Reading

Grocery Planner

Dining Out and Parties

Travel and On-the-Run Eating

Holiday Trimmings

7. How to Stay Motivated 117

It's Not All About the Food

Tasting Real Health...and Hope

Recipes 131

Symptom Tracker 192

Lifestyle Log 195

Mindful Eating Journal 197

About the Author 201

Endnotes 205

Introduction

You are here for a purpose. You have a destiny yet to be fulfilled. And to do that successfully, you need to be at your healthiest and strongest, full of energy and strength, with clear, creative thinking.

My passion is to do just that: help you be at your *very* best. It hurts my heart to see people being trapped by health challenges that can be fixed or greatly improved by making basic changes. Some changes are definitely easier than others. I know. My own health battles have made me aware of the overwhelming emotions and pain of the process.

But it is so worth it. A whole new world of freedom, health, and life is available for you—body, mind, and spirit. It changes everything.

When people find out I'm a nutritionist, the majority of them begin telling me what they ate for breakfast that day and what they had for dinner the night before. It's actually rather comical, but I want to assure you from the start that I'm not the food police. I have not always followed a clean-eating lifestyle. I have struggled with "eating right." And, I've had to allow my taste buds to change, since they used to be steeped in sugar.

I want to help you make the changes more doable. I want to help you shorten and simplify the life-changing process, by sharing secrets I've learned both personally and from my professional knowledge and experience. If I can do it as a former sugar and sweets lover, you can do it too.

We live in a busy, fast-paced world with an even shorter, 140-character attention span. To help you speed through this information and get what you need specific to your body and lifestyle, note the bolded font and feel free to skip ahead to sections that answer your most pressing questions.

You're about to discover so much more about yourself and life along this journey. It's a whole new adventure ahead. Come on; let's do it together!

Dedication

To all the beautiful ones who struggle to make health changes and who feel overwhelmed and discouraged by the seemingly monumental task of changing their eating habits.

You can still love life and enjoy food . . . even more than before. You don't have to be deprived. It can be fun and taste *incredible*. There is hope, and you *can* stay motivated.

Are you ready? Come on, let's go!

Acknowledgments

Thank you to my *dearest family and friends*, both near and far, who have been willing taste testers and a constant source of encouragement, laughs, love, support, and prayers. I treasure you so much and the precious memories we've shared, and I look forward to those yet to come! I love you dearly.

Larry and Cheryl

Thank you for countless hours of phone calls, visits, meals, and road trips. Thank you for asking the hard questions, mentoring me, and, most importantly, being a part of the deep cleaning and restoration in my life. I'm forever grateful, blessed, and changed by your love and generosity. Love you both!

Mom and Dad

None of this would have been possible without you. Your selfless, unending support and your sacrifices to help me follow my dreams still leave me speechless. It's been a wild journey with priceless memories, plenty of challenges, but lots of laughs, chocolate, and coffee. Thank you for your incredible modeling of faithfulness to me through your commitment to each other and to Him in every season. I love you so very much!

My Healer

Without You, Jesus, I wouldn't even be here journaling the pieces of the transformation You've brought to my life. Thank you for blessing the broken places in my life and for bringing me such healing, beauty, joy, and life. Thank you for making me "radiant over the goodness of the LORD."

Get ready for a journey of health empowerment. Alisha masterfully shares her own very personal story of healing in this valuable manuscript that intertwines the science of nutrition, the art of cooking and the power of spiritual health that is remarkably easy to understand, informative and practical. Alisha's credentials as a chef, dietitian and nutrition specialist were simply launching points to her pursuit for deeper understanding of the healing potential of a truly balanced lifestyle that just so happens to include great-tasting desserts! I highly recommend *Taste Radiant Living* as you pursue your own journey to health.

Dr. Rick Hall, PhD, RD
Clinical Professor and Director of Health Innovation
Arizona State University

I have admired Alisha for the many years I have known her, appreciating her entrepreneurial spirit, passion for good health, and her true understanding of living healthy and feeling healthy, not only as a certified professional, but also in her own journey. This book relates to the current difficulty in a culture focused on eating for convenience, taste, and anxiety. It's essential for help, providing a better way of eating and living, beyond just the foods that keep people stuck. Not only is the book easy to read and understand, the reader will feel their desire for health transformation is more than realistic, it's absolutely doable and lasting—no more roller coaster ups and downs or failures. Alisha more than covers this topic for a great outcome that can save years of frustration and mistakes.

Nora Ellen
Speaker – Entrepreneur – City Councilmember
Chandler, Arizona

In today's society, everyone is looking for the next gimmick, quick weight-loss solution or even to be healthy in a pill form. This is just not reality and why we find ourselves caught in a place where our health isn't a priority anymore. Our mindset must change. I believe Alisha has a Divine vision of how to give us this mindset by creating a way to simplify eating and create a realistic way to be healthy. This book is an absolute must read!

Aprile Osborne
Award-winning Realtor – Founder of five RE/MAX Franchises, South Florida – Founding Member of Equipping House
Granbury, Texas

The number one threat to our healthcare system in America is poor lifestyle choices. Alisha combines her expertise as a nutritionist with personal anecdotes to engage her readers and encourage them to make changes for a healthier and fuller life. Eating healthy *can* be simple and delicious.

Christopher Burton, MD
Speaker, Author, Coach – Executive Director
John Maxwell Team

Taste Radiant Living—a thorough, thoughtful and complete guide that will lead you to wellness and wholeness, filled with the wisdom, creativity, grace and mercy of one who has traveled the road and emerged victorious. Ask, see, follow…and surely you will experience your own transformation!

David Turner
CEO – Entrepreneur – International Christian Evangelist

From Cookie Dough to Greens: A Nutritionist's Story (How to Get Started)

Just say the words *healthy* or *vegetable* and watch a look of dread come over someone before their eyes glaze over and they drift away from the conversation. As a health professional, I've watched this happen countless times. With the bajillion diet books, websites, and blogs, the reality shows, and the latest fad diets, information overload easily creates confusion. *Healthy*—what exactly does this term mean? Somehow, our culture has found it easy to equate being healthy with an image of misery, boredom, and tasteless, cardboard-textured foods. Being healthy is something we all want but aren't sure we're willing to pay the price to get. I know. I've struggled through these questions and challenges myself. I actually used to think that I ate "healthy" (even as a nutrition graduate student and a newly-trained dietitian), until my own health challenges forced me to reexamine what I had been taught about being "healthy."

With the changing political and economic times and the health-care crises all around us, from obesity, heart disease, diabetes, and cancer, to rapidly changing healthcare and insurance systems, it's urgent for us to take responsibility for our health. This includes everything from making changes you've been dreading because of a current diagnosis, to shedding a few extra pounds, to preventing future health challenges, to living the healthiest, most energetic life possible. It's time to take the next steps on the journey to health in order to learn how to get and stay well. You don't have the luxury of time or money to be sick and tired. Life is too short. *Now* is the time to be well, so that your health doesn't hold you back from living life. It's time for your most fulfilling and prosperous days to be lived.

I love sweets—chocolate to be specific. During most of my childhood years (OK, all of my life), holidays, times with family and friends, and even my personal interests all centered around food. My "sweet tooth" came through my family line. I take after my paternal Grandpa most closely; he *always* had a little candy bowl with Hershey's kisses and other delectable treats by his favorite chair. My sweet Grandma also fostered my sweet tooth, as she constantly kept the cookie jar full of her freshly baked cookies. My maternal Grandma passed on the most amazing sweet bread (*potica* from Yugoslavia), cinnamon rolls, and other made-from-scratch pies, cakes, and cookies, which were always special holiday and everyday traditions. I guess you can say sweets were in my blood.

My first cooking exploits began early, and thankfully, film captured the memories. At two years old, I stood on a chair in order to reach the counter, wearing my little pink footie pajamas, confidently mixing cornbread batter. My kitchen adventures progressed from frosting Grandma's sugar cookies in my red frilly dress to proudly displaying my Easy-Bake Oven, which cooked miniature desserts by the heat of a light bulb, with my first little, double chocolate layer cake. These humble beginnings continued as I joined 4-H in fourth grade, where I entered my goods in the Arizona Pima County Fair. Of course, mine were *all* desserts, and they all contained chocolate. (All three won Best of Class, by the way). Making chocolate chip cookies (and dough) on Sunday afternoons became my favorite weekly tradition, where the dough was as much of a treat as the cookies. In fact, my frozen dough logs were meant to be sliced and baked, but they rarely made it onto a cookie sheet. Between winning more "Best of Class" ribbons for my family dessert recipes in Ohio's Greene County Fair and indulging in nightly bedtime goodies, I continued to grow more passionate about baking and sweets.

By the time I reached college, I knew a degree in nutrition would be the perfect fit. Nutrition incorporated my love of being in the kitchen with my fascination and desire to promote health and wellness, with a better match for my squeamishness than direct hands-on care. Ironically, my love of desserts fit amazingly well with the no-fat/low-fat fad of the 90s. I could easily tweak my recipes to reduce the fat . . . or not! I breezed through college, thinking, "I'm thankful that I've always eaten healthily." I continued to do so (or so I thought) as I fueled my busy days with pasta, bagels, frozen yogurt, sweets, and diet Dr Pepper®.

After finishing my master's degree in nutrition and completing my registration as a dietitian, I finally got my wake-up call—literally. I woke up one morning with my heart racing. I spent the day at the emergency room, with heart monitors showing my heartbeat to be a near constant 140 beats per minute. Needless to say, it did not feel good. Thus began my journey to true health.

My health had seemingly been fine up until then, although I grew up with a "sensitive" stomach that was upset easily by fast food and heavy, rich foods. But I was healthy, other than allergies and an odd phase in junior high and high school when big, itchy, red hives erupted over my entire body and even my lips. (This was quite attractive for a sixteen-year-old!) The allergist suspected food allergies, so I went for a brief time without strawberries and corn (which is in *everything*), but thankfully, the hives soon cleared.

I was super sick with mono right before my senior year of high school. Amidst emotional goodbyes to lifelong friends and family members, packing boxes, and loading a U-Haul to move from Arizona to Virginia, I was miserable. I slept most of five days traveling across the country and for most of another week during the unloading and settling in to our new home. I was down a full month, but took several more weeks to regain energy. In fact, I don't think my health was ever quite the same through college.

Then the stress of college had me taking daily Mylanta doses for a "nervous" stomach. But that was normal, right? It was no big deal to me at the time. Unfortunately, adult cystic acne began near the end of college, requiring cortisone shots in the deeply inflamed nickel-sized lumps on my face. The day I had to have eight injections, I figured something needed to change. So, I began daily antibiotics (erythromycin) for a couple of years, as it helped both my stomach and my skin—or so it seemed.

I pushed through graduate school in nineteen months, completing a 900+ hour internship (working forty-plus hours a week . . . for free!) while completing and defending my thesis at the same time. I was starting to experience more fatigue and increasing stomach issues, apparently stemming from food allergies. I reduced problematic foods, but kept going at high speed. The cystic acne began to worsen again. This time, it was devastating. At one time, I counted up to twenty painful cysts on my face on the same day. This timing was by no means ideal, as wedding season was in full swing for my friends. I certainly didn't feel very photogenic as a bridesmaid or wedding assistant.

Finally, everything culminated when I returned from a vacation in Italy with a horrible flu. I couldn't keep food down for seven days, requiring my first emergency room trip for fluids. I lost ten pounds that week, which I really didn't have to lose. I hadn't fully recovered from the illness before experiencing some other major family health challenges. About that same time, my Grandpa suffered a stroke, resulting in some left-sided paralysis, and within a month, my mom's car was hit by a drunk driver while she was stopped at a red light. Thankfully, she only initially suffered whiplash, but within weeks this flared into fibromyalgia. Then came my awful wake-up call.

With the second ER trip for my racing pulse, my crazy symptoms resulted in a three-month medical leave from work. I could sleep ten to twelve hours a night and still wake up feeling like I had been hit by a train. I continued to run a low-grade fever for about three months, along with the racing heartbeat, heart palpitations, stomach discomfort, and the dreaded cystic acne. I was miserable.

Over the next several months, I had numerous tests, including a radioactive iodine uptake test on my thyroid, tons of bloodwork, a cardiac stress test, thirty days with a heart monitor, an upper GI test, and more. A high TSH (thyroid-stimulating hormone) was the only out-of-range result throughout the testing, and this typically coincides with a *slower* pulse, not a racing pulse. Finally, after two years with no answers and a milder recurrence of symptoms, my primary doctor diagnosed me with chronic fatigue syndrome and sent me home with a prescription for an antidepressant, telling me that I would deal with this for the rest of my life.

Something in me rose up that day and said, "This is ridiculous! There has to be something more I can do." Of course I was depressed to some extent. What 27-year-old wouldn't be if she could hardly work ten to twenty hours per week and barely function beyond the essentials of life—all while still dealing with cystic acne? (As a side note, I had refused the acne drugs my dermatologist wanted me to take, as I had no desire to be on the birth control that was required with the medication. I figured if it wasn't safe for a pregnant mom with a developing baby, how could it be good for my own body?) Questions began turning in my mind: What really is health? What is healing? How do I get and maintain it? Does what I'm eating *really* matter *that much*? What have I been taught about health? Why isn't it working? In the remaining pages, I'll answer these questions and share the rich, life-changing lessons and principles I discovered during this season of my life.

How do you begin? **Decide to get started**. Come on a journey with me! Partner with me as your coach in the next few pages. I'll take you back to the basics of nutrition and give you tips on how to simplify "healthy," which can result in you losing some unwanted pounds, improving your overall wellness, reducing a host of pesky symptoms you may be experiencing, improving your digestive issues, clearing your skin, and boosting your immunity and energy. I'll introduce you to ways of making a healthy lifestyle taste so good, you—and your family and friends—can actually enjoy it. If I can do it as a former cookie-dough lover who had never had (or cared to have) kale, you can do it too. Read and practice the simple tips in the pages ahead, and watch as the results come more quickly than you ever thought possible!

2

"Healthy" Gets a Makeover: How to Get Motivated

Forget the Die-t—Start the Lifestyle!

I hate diets. Just the word *diet* brings dread and a grimace. It sounds so restrictive and painful—you can see the three-letter word built right into it! For a lot of people, a new year or season prompts them to "buck up," thinking, "This time, this diet is going to work." You and I both know what happens next. You make it for a few days, or maybe a month at most, and then you're back to the same old same old. Nothing really changed, except you feel like you've failed yet again at another "die-t."

This cycle of serial dieting simply sets us up for failure. Even worse, it has created a bad rap for the word *healthy*, making us believe that healthy food is entirely boring and tasteless, and will make us feel deprived and miserable.

Without a change in our perspective, we will continue to perceive *healthy* negatively, and no changes will be made, while we'll continue experiencing the same results. This is the true definition of insanity: doing the same thing over and over while expecting different results. **Real change must begin from within, and true**

motivation begins with a new mindset. An ancient proverb says, "What you think, you become." And it's true!

Thoughts → Beliefs → Words → Actions → Habits
→ Future and Destiny

We must get a fresh taste and perspective on being healthy, so we can get the results we really want.

So, how about a new approach? What if the diet thing dies forever and transitions into a *lifestyle*? A lifestyle is a regular part of life. A new habit. A new way of living. A daily thing. The new normal. **When we adjust our lifestyle, we become free to stop focusing on what we *can't have*, start focusing on what our body actually *needs* for wellness**, and begin enjoying the almost immediate effects of a more nourished body.

Based on my professional experience, it's much easier to prevent and maintain well-being than to regain it. In addition to my own challenges, I've worked with clients facing extremes, from being on life-supporting kidney dialysis and battling terminal cancer, to those wanting to lose a few pounds and put an end to annoying symptoms, to those dealing with minor and severe food sensitivities, and those working to stop pre-diabetes. It's especially hard to watch those in later stages of a disease, wondering if the results could have been entirely different had changes been made earlier. But, I understand. It's easy to think that what you're eating doesn't really matter. Hind sight is always 20/20, and "coulda, shoulda, woulda" can't change it. Early in life, it seems like what you're eating can't possibly affect you. But in the end, many of my clients wish they would have made changes much earlier. As in my case, many of us just didn't know any different. The American food culture, from eating traditions, grocery stores, and media ads to our medical system with little-to-no nutritional training, has programmed us to make the disconnect between our food and our health. For instance, one dear lady I worked with was able to manage her diabetes in as little as a month with some simple eating changes. At her follow-up, she said with tears in her eyes, "Why didn't my doctor tell me this?"

Thankfully, your health no longer needs to be in jeopardy from of lack of knowledge. Thought it's easy to ignore current health information, statistics and trends, or even to delay personal health check-ups, choosing not to deal with health challenges or symptoms, **being informed is a huge piece of changing your perspective. Knowledge increases power!** When we know the potential outcome if current patterns don't change, we're empowered with options for course corrections that can lead us to a better end.

I was not alone in facing my body's challenges, and I'm still not. America is facing a health-care crisis. Just look at those you know and love. It's likely that you know someone (or several) dealing with heart disease, diabetes, cancer, yo-yo dieting, weight struggles, an eating disorder, gluten sensitivity, a food allergy, digestive concerns, autism . . . the list goes on. The rates of these conditions have mushroomed at astonishing rates over the last few years, and conditions found primarily in textbooks are now popping up all around us. Check out these statistics on **the state of America's health** and what it's costing us:

- "Chronic diseases and conditions—such as **heart disease, stroke, cancer, diabetes, obesity, and arthritis**—are among the ***most common, costly and preventable of all health problems***."[1]

- In 2012, approximately **50 percent of all US adults** (117 million) have one or more chronic health conditions; 25 percent of adults have two or more.[2]
- About **47 percent of adults have at least one major risk factor for heart disease or stroke**: uncontrolled high blood pressure, uncontrolled high LDL cholesterol, or are current smokers. [3]
- Seven of the top ten causes of death in 2010 were chronic diseases. **Heart disease and cancer together accounted for nearly half** (48 percent) of all deaths.
- **Eighty-six percent of all health-care spending** in 2006 was **for the 50 percent of the population** who have one or more chronic medical conditions.[4]

❖ Obesity is a serious health concern. In 2012, the Center for Disease Control (CDC) reported that **69 percent** of US adults over the age of twenty **were overweight** and **35 percent were obese**.[5, 6]

- Health-care experts project that by 2030, **86 percent of adults will be overweight** and **50 percent will be obese**.[7]
- **Obesity increases the risk of a host of medical complications** (as many as thirty), including type 2 diabetes, high blood pressure, cancer, heart disease, gallbladder disease, arthritis, sleep apnea, and many more.

- Weight-related health problems are now being **diagnosed in children,** with **17 percent** between the ages of two and nineteen being obese in 2012.[8]
- Direct **health-care costs for obesity run 42% higher** than for those at healthy weights. Currently, medical costs range from $147 to $210 billion yearly in 2009, and are projected to reach 21 percent of our total health-care costs by 2018.[9, 10, 11]
- Having **one obese person** in a family **causes an extra 8 percent of the family income** to be spent on healthcare.[12]

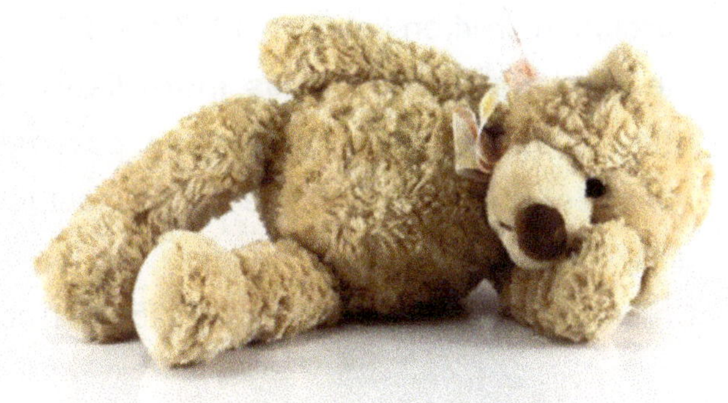

Bear-y sad state-of-health

❖ In 2012, the Center for Disease Control reported that **9 percent** of the population had been **diagnosed with diabetes** (though nearly 25 percent of diabetics are actually undiagnosed). **One in three are prediabetic**, yet the majority of these (nine out of ten) are unaware of this.[13, 14]

- **Diabetic complications are the leading cause of kidney disease, non-accident-related amputations, and blindness, as well as two to four times higher risk of heart disease**.
- Seventy-one percent of diabetics have high blood pressure, and 60 to 70 percent have some form of neuropathy (nerve damage and disorders).[15, 16]
- **Medical costs** for diabetics are **2.3 times higher** than nondiabetics.[17, 18]

❖ **Food allergies** affect 4 percent of adults and 8 percent of children, meaning as many as **one in thirteen children**, or about two in every classroom.[19, 20]

- The CDC reports that food allergies have **increased 50 percent** in children between 1997 and 2011, making the kids **two to four times more likely to have other related conditions (asthma, eczema, other allergies)** compared to those kids without food allergies.[21, 22, 23]
- Children's food allergies cost nearly $25 billion per year.[24]

❖ **Celiac disease** affects three million people in America (approximately 1 percent), with a diagnosis rate of **1 in 133**, but rates are projected to reach 50 to 60 percent by 2019.[25, 26]

- Another **eighteen to twenty-two million consumers eat gluten-free** to manage gluten sensitivity, while another **twelve million classified themselves as "gluten-intolerant"** and also avoid gluten.[27]

- **Autism rates** have increased 30 percent from 2008 to 2010, and have doubled since 2000 (partially due to increased awareness and diagnostic criteria). **One in sixty-eight children** are currently diagnosed as being on the autism spectrum.[28, 29]

- A *Journal of the American Medical Association* **study reports medical care** (drug errors and side effects, hospital infections, etc.) **as the third leading cause of death**.[30]

Let me clarify this last statistic about medical care. Unfortunately, errors in medical care are a reality. This is not at all a disparagement of our medical system, but we must face the truth about the state of our country's health. Usually, we are quick to rely on a doctor or medication to solve our problems. But the **majority of medications simply treat symptoms and do not address the root cause**. Additionally, it is common to be on several medications at once, increasing the likelihood of drug interactions and side effects. Even TV bombards us with over-the-counter and prescription drug ads, growing more than any other ad category in the last four years, exceeding $6 billion in 2016.[31] This strategy of the pharmaceutical companies complicates everything: increasing drug costs and healthcare spending, suggesting high-priced and limited-use medications, promoting fear of conditions (and even promoting "new conditions"), glossing over serious side effects, and distracting doctor-patient appointments to discussing marketing tactics instead of the most beneficial and relevant health information.[32]

Additionally, doctors, nurses, practitioners, pharmacists, and other healthcare professionals are people who, though well-trained, can make mistakes and have limits to their abilities. Even worse, **errors in surgeries or even simple procedures occur**. Our culture tends to put them on a pedestal, as though they have all the answers and are perfect. I'm so grateful that we have their knowledge and expertise, especially in crisis situations, but we simply cannot place all our hope for a healthy future on them. Our medical system is about to change drastically, and we may be in for a shock. We're already experiencing much higher insurance premiums, co-pays, and prescription costs, shorter appointments, and unhappy (and fewer) physicians due to new regulations and more red tape. **How many medications (and resulting interactions), procedures (some of which result in errors), and high healthcare costs could be prevented with simple lifestyle changes and better nutrition?**

Here are a few more numbers from a 2011 CDC report that show us the **top four health risk behaviors**, which are the main causes of illness and premature death related to chronic diseases and conditions:

- lack of exercise or physical activity
- alcohol abuse
- poor nutrition
- tobacco use

Take a look at the first two of these lifestyle risk factors. The numbers are sobering:

- Physical Activity
  - **Fifty-two percent** of adults over eighteen **did not meet recommended aerobic exercise** or **physical activity levels**, and **76 percent did not meet recommendations for muscle-strengthening activities** based on the *2008 Federal Physical Activity Guidelines for Americans.*[33]
  - Only one in three adults participate in the recommended amount of physical activity weekly, with **less than 5 percent of adults exercising just thirty minutes each day**.[34, 35]
  - Only **one in three children are physically active every day**. Rather, children spend *seven hours on average in front of a screen every day.*[36, 37]

- Poor Nutrition
  - **Ninety percent of Americans consume too much sodium**, increasing their risk of high blood pressure. Reducing sodium by just 1,200 milligrams per day could save up to $20 billion a year in medical costs.[38]
  - **Less than 18 percent** of adults in each state **consumed the recommended amount of fruit, and less than 14 percent consumed the recommended amount of vegetables**, based on the 2015 *Behavioral Risk Factor Surveillance System Report* by the CDC.
    - This means **82 percent do *not*** eat the recommended servings of fruit, and **85 percent do *not*** eat the recommended servings of vegetables.[39, 40]

- The numbers for children are even more concerning, with **60 percent consuming fewer fruit servings** than recommended, and **93 percent consuming fewer vegetable servings** than recommended.[41]

So, what *are* we eating? A 2005's *US News & World Report* article, "One Sweet Nation" shows **we're eating an incredible amount of sugar**.[42] The 2016 USDA's *Food Commodity Consumption* report shows that from 2007-2008, the average American total vegetable consumption was 162 pounds per year, with only 1.42 cups consumed daily. The top 3 vegetables consumed included potatoes (52 pounds), tomatoes (30.5 pounds) and lettuce (13.8 pounds), with French fries and pizza being the top contributors to these veggie leaders. The annual fruit consumption from the same period was 119 pounds per person, with only 1.05 cups consumed daily. Of this 119 pounds, nearly 40% was in the form of a processed, refined juice: 16 pounds of apple juice and 31 pounds (just over 3 gallons) of orange juice. The following chart shows this large contrast in the types and amounts of our yearly food intake. [43]

Food	Pounds per Year Consumed by the Average Adult
Sugar	142
High-fructose corn syrup	61
Soft drinks	53 gallons
Potatoes	52
Tomatoes	30.5
Lettuce – Romaine and Iceberg	13.8
Apples	11.6
Fresh oranges	3
Bananas	11.6[44, 45]

With my love of sweets, I can see how we easily hit these numbers! It's no wonder **0.5% of our food budget is spent on green leafy veggies and 4% on fruit, while 17% is spent on refined grain items and nearly 15% on sugar and candies**, according to the *USDA's Economic Research Service's* report on expenditure from 1998-2006.[46] Sadly, much of the time, we've moved far away from eating real, whole foods in their natural state, instead choosing manufactured foods: items that have been processed, stripped of naturally occurring nutrients and fiber that are vital to health, filled with refined sugars, treated with additional chemicals to increase their shelf life, and colorized to make them look appetizing. Look at a package and try reading the ingredient lists. Can you pronounce the ingredients? Do you even know what they are? Your body probably doesn't either.

Take a minute to observe what is being purchased and consumed when you're at the mall, grocery store, work, or out to eat. You can see exactly what the consumption statistics and budget spending numbers are saying. They tell a story that clearly indicates how we have failed to prioritize our health and take necessary care of our bodies. It is astonishing to think that on the average, only about 3 percent of adults achieve the four simple habits for health previously listed. **Something must change if we want to see different results in our country over the next decades**. We have already seen drastic changes in the last twenty-five to thirty years. Can you imagine what the state of health could be like for our children and grandchildren if things continue unchanged?

We must, must, must start taking responsibility for our health. Of these top seven chronic conditions (and causes of mortality), **five are preventable with nutrition and lifestyle changes**. **How much of what we're facing as a country is caused by what we are (or are not) eating**, and how we are (or are not) taking care of our bodies? Prevention is no longer an option; it is absolutely *essential*!

Strangely enough, around the globe, nutritionists are observing the first generation battling obesity *and* malnutrition simultaneously. **We've so filled our bodies with poor-quality, processed, empty-calorie foods that we've added on excess weight, while at the same time starving our bodies of real, true nutrition** (i.e., vitamins, minerals, antioxidants) that are needed for cell, organ, and biochemical processes to function properly. The BBC published the results of the International Food Policy Research Institute's *2016 Global Nutrition Report*, stating that 44 percent of countries now have "very serious levels" of both undernutrition and obesity. Further, the report states "hundreds of millions of people are malnourished because they are overweight, as well as having too much sugar, salt or cholesterol in their blood." The research co-chairman, Lawrence Haddad, put it this way: "We now live in a world where being malnourished is the new normal." Though we often think of being malnourished as a state of starvation, it includes all forms of poor or improper nutrition. With one in three people suffering from some form of malnutrition in this 129-country study, being malnourished is becoming a huge challenge globally with the rise in obesity.[47]

Epigenetics, a newer field of science, explores how **DNA—or our genes—can be altered by everything from social, cultural, and emotional factors to lifestyle factors, including exercise and nutrition**. Literally, gene expression can be turned on and off by these and other factors. It's fascinating to think that we can have this much of an influence over our health rather than just being a product of our genetics. Moms-to-be, this gives you a unique opportunity to significantly influence your baby's health during (and before) pregnancy. (Fathers, don't think your eating has no effect though; your impact just has less research behind it.) Studies have shown that preconception eating can affect your child's—and even your grandchildren's—genetics long-term, influencing risk factors of diabetes, obesity, and other chronic diseases according to research reviews by neuroscientist Dr. Caroline Leaf.[48]

The changes have to start with us personally. As we begin to make the transitions in our own lives for ourselves and for those we love, the health revolution can begin, impacting the health of our workplaces, schools, communities, cities, states, and country, and that of the generations to come. Sounds easy, right? Well, it really can be, and I'm going to show you how. So, let's get started!

Before moving on to some specific applications, I want to focus on one of the most important personal motivators. Besides the sheer numbers being a motivation, I want you to take a few minutes to get a really clear vision of what "good health" will look like for you. What do you want? What exactly will this look like? What clothing/styles will you be able to wear? How much energy will you have? How will your lab results improve? What symptoms will disappear? How much muscle tone would you like to gain? How about your endurance levels?

I'm serious; this is that important. **Without a vision or a dream, discipline and motivation will be nonexistent.** Without a vision, we can run rather directionless, not knowing what we are running toward. Without knowing what you are working to achieve, you won't have the motivation to make the better choices. So, before skipping on to the next chapter, write out what your health goals and vision specifically look like. (See the end of the chapter for the goal sheet.)

Now that we have concluded it's time for dieting to end, we can have real hope for changing our health. **Perspective is everything.** Often, a little tweak can make a big difference. Here are a few starter tips to help you set your focus and achieve your goals:

1. **Make this a journey.** Habits don't usually change overnight. Give yourself some grace and enjoy the process to discover what works best for you. Even your taste buds need some time to adjust to flavors other than very sweet and very salty to which they are typically programmed.
2. **Make this a food adventure.** Discover new foods, new recipes, new flavors, and new favorites. You will be surprised by how many foods and flavors you have to work with, and by how amazingly delicious they actually are! (And by how many veggies are out there besides iceberg lettuce, potatoes, tomatoes, and corn.)
3. **Look for the beauty in real food.** We've become so accustomed to processed, lifeless, dull-colored food that we've

What are your goals for your health?

Be sure to make them *measurable* (put a specific number and time to it), *achievable* (you want to maintain a level of success to keep you motivated), and *realistic* (push yourself, but not for impossible results).

Short-term goals:

1.

2.

3.

Long-term goals:

1.

2.

3.

3

How (and What to Eat) to Make Healthy Delicious

"Alisha, you must stop sugar and dairy," he said in broken English with a thick Chinese accent.

No! I screamed inwardly, as I listened to the words of the first natural (and 100 percent traditional Chinese) health practitioner I visited for the host of miserable symptoms I was experiencing. How was I *possibly* going to make these changes? I loved chocolate, sweets, and cheese; sugar and dairy were my food foundation. What was I going to eat? But from the current state of my body, I also knew I had nothing to lose, except possibly the fatigue, acne, upset stomach, and misery—*if* he was right!

So, my new eating lifestyle began. Even with an advanced degree in nutrition *and* registered dietitian credentials, I had heard nothing in any of my lectures about dairy or even moderate sugar intakes affecting health. At the time, natural sweeteners were still on the fringe, and alternative dairy products were even more foreign to me and rare to find. I had never shopped at any grocery store other than the major chains, which carried virtually no "natural" foods at the time. My new eating lifestyle was boring, bland, frustratingly restrictive, and monotonous. I really missed my favorite breads, carbs, and sweets and the veggies weren't very exciting . . . until I started to notice changes. I started feeling better, and the acne became less inflamed, with cysts forming less frequently as I reduced sugar, dairy, and highly- refined wheat. Could certain foods really have been affecting my body that much?

With that, I began to delve further into new food possibilities, determined to make what my body needed taste better and find a few treats that wouldn't send my body back into overload. I expanded my grocery-shopping options and started spending more time in the kitchen with *real* food instead of sweets. I began to study other "food lifestyles" than the ones I'd been taught about in school, which usually revolved around processed, sugary supplement drinks and eating patterns based primarily on grains, pastas, and breads. Some of my friends were very committed to the raw foods trend, so I checked it out. It seemed extreme, but I was desperate to have my health back. In the end, it made perfect sense. Why wouldn't our bodies heal when given the right building blocks? Even a cut on the finger demonstrates the simple concept that we were naturally made to heal.

I learned by trial and error. Slowly, I moved away from my favorite foods like cookie dough, pasta, doughy bagels, and sugary frozen yogurt to a plant-based lifestyle, packed with nutrition that would allow my body to heal and rebuild. I made smoothies. I juiced. I made fresh almond milk. I ate salads—a *lot* of salads—and I also found other ways to be creative and get in my daily veggies. I made my own salad dressings. I made my own "new desserts," experimenting with natural sweeteners and other flavors, like lemon, pumpkin, fruit, and pure chocolate. Life was beginning to be fun again . . . and it tasted great! My body was not craving the same empty-calorie sweets anymore.

For me, this was a several-year process that I continued to adjust according to the seasons of my life, though it eventually settled into a nice balance. You name it, I've probably tried it: no sugar, no dairy, no wheat, no gluten, raw foods, juicing, vegan, vegetarian, high protein, candida diets, cleanses, and more. With each, I saw benefits. My body began to heal. My energy, digestion, and skin were improving. In fact, even though I am fair-skinned with red hair and burn easily with sun exposure, I began to tan beautifully during my juicing days. With my skin saturated with nutrients, I had natural sun protection *and* it gave me the most amazing tan! This made me a believer.

Before you close the book, thinking you'll have to endure the same frustrations and trial-and-error misery I faced on my journey, **I want to share the things I've learned that can short-cut your health makeover.**

While we approach "healthy" from new angles, let's start by making it about the **food that you *can* have** rather than what you *can't* have. When did we start limiting our food choices to manufactured and engineered items? In America, we have food in abundance. It's bountiful, plentiful (in most areas), and flavorful. It's colorful and, most importantly, nutrient dense. A simple look at **Nutrition 101 shows us what our bodies need to be fueled correctly**, taking us back to the basics. Here's also a look at the "why" behind nutrition so you can learn, increase your power, and even begin to enjoy and crave these essentials for your body.

Set the Foundation

Food provides us with the **building blocks for life, energy, and healing**. The body runs according to what goes in it. For this, we have two primary choices: "live" foods or "dead" foods.

- ❖ **Live food**—This does not mean you need to grow your own food supply, eat straight from your garden, or eat everything raw, uncooked, and crunchy. But when we consume foods as **close to their natural state as possible, more of the nutrition is available in a useable form for the body**. Look what our bodies have to gain:
    - **Nutrient-dense foods protect, nourish, and heal** the body, and contain higher amounts of:
        - **Vitamins and minerals**, which are essential compounds in our food (not usually made by the body, or produced by the body in limited quantities) required for body functions and processes, metabolism, energy production, growth, and even structural components (bones and teeth).
        - **Antioxidants and phytonutrients**, which prevent oxidation. Think of a sliced apple turning brown. These nutrient powerhouses prevent "oxidative stress" (the "browning" damage by harmful substances), and ultimately work to protect cells, organs, and tissues from disease, damage, the environment, and aging. These are often identified by their color (reds, blues, purples, oranges, yellows, greens, and whites). Typically, the darker the color, the better. Researchers are just now

identifying and studying *thousands* of these plant components that work to strengthen the immune system, reduce the risk of cancer and heart disease, protect vision, strengthen blood vessels, prevent aging, and build strong skin, cells, tissue, and organs. The list goes on and on! The bottom line is that the more of these antioxidants and phytonutrients you consume regularly, the healthier you'll be.

  - **Fiber**, which traps and binds toxins (cholesterol and metabolic wastes), preventing reabsorption back into the body, and assisting with bulk removal of these wastes from the body. It also regulates blood sugars, maintains healthy body weight, promotes digestive health, and keeps us feeling full between meals. Your goal should be to consume thirty to forty grams per day; unfortunately, most people average only about sixteen grams per day.[49]

- All these nutrient-dense options are especially found in plant sources: **fruits, vegetables, beans, nuts, and seeds**.
- They bring life and energy, keep body systems functioning, build the immune system, protect the body, remove toxins, and help regulate your weight.

❖ **Dead food**— The majority of grocery stores, restaurants, and fast-food chains capitalize on highly-processed convenience foods, which are a huge part of the average American diet.

- Provides little nutritional value. Simply put, the nutrition has been stripped away, leaving an **empty-calorie product with low to no vitamins, minerals, antioxidants, fiber, or phytonutrients**.
- **Lowers energy** levels and compromises the body due to lack of nutrients.
- **Increases risk factors** and the **body's vulnerability to disease** as a result of poor, nutrient-depleted content.
- Is found concentrated in **canned and packaged snack foods, sugary beverages, cereals, prepackaged meals, fast food, and frozen dinners**.
- Often leads to **weight gain**, as the body stores away excess simple sugars and calories and protects itself from unnatural substances (food additives, preservatives, etc.) by "walling them off" and packing them away in fat cells.

Make It Colorful

Who would have guessed that many of the health problems rampant in America are actually linked to malnutrition? Living in a wealthy nation, we don't think of Americans as being malnourished, but this is often the case. Our amazingly strong and uniquely designed bodies adapt for a while, but they can only take so much nutrient deprivation before healthy body processes and pathways break down, toxins build up, and symptoms begin to surface. Fascinatingly, many of our cravings are actually the body's way of crying out for more nutrition, not just empty calories. Looking back, I believe this was my primary nutritional issue, as "dead food" outweighed the "live food," and my body was missing the nutrient-dense goodness it needed.

Live foods need to be the focus to nourish and rebuild the body. This becomes **a lifestyle emphasizing a colorful variety of plant-rich, minimally processed whole foods**. This doesn't mean you have to be vegetarian or vegan. As noted earlier, Americans severely lack adequate nutrition, with only 14 to 18 percent of adults hitting the goal of five servings of produce daily. Current studies by nonprofit educational research groups (e.g., the Harvard School of Public Health) and numerous medical professionals recommend an even higher number of produce servings, encouraging a **minimum of seven (and up to thirteen) servings of fruits and vegetables daily**.[50, 51, 52, 53]

Research shows that the nutrient density of vitamins, minerals, antioxidants, and fiber found in fruits and vegetables specifically lowers blood pressure and protects against cancers, heart disease and stroke, diabetes, digestive disorders, degeneration in vision (cataracts), Alzheimer's, and other declines associated with aging.[54, 55, 56] A recent University College of London study in the September 2014 edition of the *Journal of Epidemiology and Community Health* reports that **eating seven or more vegetable and fruit servings per day reduces the risks of cancer deaths by 25 percent and risks of heart disease deaths by 31 percent.** The study also found that vegetables have significantly higher health benefits than fruits do, but each added serving brings benefits, reducing the risk of death *by any cause*: one to three servings of fruits and veggies by 14 percent, three to five servings by 29 percent, five to seven servings by 36 percent, **with seven or more servings bringing a whopping 42 percent reduction**.[57, 58]

A **plant-rich** emphasis also **consists of nuts, seeds, beans, legumes, whole grains, fresh oils, herbs, and spices, and reasonable portions of lean meats**. The possibilities are endless, and they're beautiful. The produce aisles contain some of the most *brilliantly colored, bursting-with-flavor* foods in existence!

It is doable, and following a plant-rich diet doesn't mean eating salads all day. I'll show you how as we move forward. Just wait!

Build Strength and Structure

In order to have a strong foundation, we must build strength and structure, which come from the following:

- **Protein**—Protein is required not only for muscle, but also for the structure and function of cells, and for the regulation of the body's tissues (hair, nails, skin), organs, body systems, and immunity.
  - Primary sources: **poultry, fish, beef, beans, and nuts**

  I'm going to simplify the often sensitive, emotional, and controversial debate on protein by saying **it is essential**! I've seen strict, plant-based vegetarian and vegan diets be successful, *but usually just for a short time*. During the season I was eating vegan and primarily raw foods, my body initially experienced great benefits. But then, I began developing complications, as I needed more protein and calories to be functioning optimally and for healing and rebalancing. While Americans tend to eat way too much meat, meat is not the main culprit. Rather, filling up on sugar and other processed foods, and not eating enough nutrient-dense produce (veggies and fruit) and other important plant-rich selections (such as nuts, beans, and healthy oils) are the main problems.

Sadly, many vegetarians and vegans are among some of the sickest people I have worked with professionally. Typically, they are not getting enough calories, protein, and/or they are deficient in other nutrients usually supplied by animal-based foods. Though people choose this lifestyle with the best intentions, it is challenging and quite time-consuming to eat vegan or vegetarian in our culture. It must be done correctly to keep the body in balance and avoid deficiencies. Unfortunately, simply replacing protein with refined carbs, breads, wheat, soy and other vegetarian items will not lead to health.

The recent rise in popularity of the vegetarian and vegan lifestyles is partly due to the awareness of what's *really* in our standard American food, including everything from hormones, additives, preservatives, pesticides, and GMOs (genetically modified organisms). Vegetarianism and veganism are also supported by the exposure of the often inhumane practices used to create, package, and process meat products. Much of this info comes through documentaries, some of which are great exposés, but many lack accurate research, present concepts through emotional filters, and often incite fear in viewers.

The rise in these eating lifestyles is also often related to spirituality. Vegetarianism and veganism can attach themselves to religions and worldviews that seem to be full of light, life, and love. In truth, these religions subtly open doors to powers of darkness, which affect health and much more over time. In more extreme cases, I've also seen them form a religion in their system of beliefs and rules. The truth is that food doesn't increase our spirituality, but rather is a form of nourishment and a source of enjoyment. Our food choices should be a reflection of our values and beliefs in the One who is the only *Source* of Life, Love, and Peace. As we choose to believe Truth and treasure our *true* identities, our food choices will be ones that most benefit our bodies and take care of the world around us.

❖ **Fat**—Fat serves as an energy source, keeps you feeling full longer, and is a requirement for the absorption of some vitamins. Fat is also a main component of our brain, glands, organs, hormones, and cell membranes.

- Primary sources: **nuts, seeds, avocados, olives, cold-water fish, and cold-pressed oils**

The type of fat plays an important role in how well each cell functions, and thus, the efficiency of how each organ and body system performs. Will the cells be flexible, moving about freely and allowing nutrients in and wastes out? Or will they be rigid, trapping toxins and functioning poorly?

Without enough "good" fats, health will deteriorate. The key is to reduce and even eliminate the "bad" fats, and to add in the "good" fats with the proper balance. The low-fat, fat-free days of the past are over. Fats are truly essential! Your body needs them for structure, function, energy, and weight maintenance.

Here are the main types of fats and oils that we eat and how they work in the body:

Unsaturated Fats—Unsaturated oils are "good fats" known for their healthful benefits. Their unique structure keeps them liquid at room temperature.

– Primary sources: **olives, nuts, seeds, avocados**

Olive oil is one of the most common sources. As part of the Mediterranean food culture, it's known for heart-health benefits, but it comes loaded with antioxidants and phytonutrients, also believed to help regulate nearly 100 genes associated with communication between cells, age-related processes, and especially with lowering inflammation. Its well-researched and all-around powerful, protective benefits work to:

- Protect against heart disease, high blood pressure, and strokes
- Prevent blood clot formation
- Reduce cholesterol and LDLs
- Lower inflammation (and inflammatory markers)
- Lower blood sugars, helping defend against diabetes
- Protect bone health, preventing osteoporosis
- Prevent cancer, especially breast, respiratory tract, and digestive tract
- Guard against age-related diseases: Alzheimer's, osteoporosis, skin aging
- Protect against rheumatoid arthritis and restore mobility and joint use in diagnosed patients
- Extend longevity (lowering the overall risk of death from all health-related causes)[59, 60]

Extra virgin olive oil (EVOO) that is cold-pressed or expeller-pressed gives the most benefits. Look for organic varieties sold in dark bottles that is stored in cool areas, as heat and light breakdown the valuable, protective nutrients.

Omega-3s—essential fatty acids that our body can't produce on its own. These unsaturated oils known for their **anti-inflammatory properties** are required for **brain development and function, chronic disease prevention** and much more:

- Can lower pain levels
- Reduce inflammation
- Raise HDL and lower LDL
- Decrease blood pressure
- Help prevent blood clots
- Improve blood sugar
- Protect vision and fight dry eyes
- Help maintain mental clarity with aging
- Support brain development in children
- Can regulate and stabilize behavioral, attention, and emotional disorders
- Help stabilize and improve moods
- Slow and prevent cancer growth
- Help balance hormone levels
- Improve skin health

Omega-6s—good sources of unsaturated plant oils. They are more beneficial than high levels of saturated fats, but in **high, imbalanced amounts can make the body more likely to experience**:

- Blood clot formation and sticky blood cells
- Thicker blood
- Blood vessel constriction and spasms (higher blood pressure)
- Inflammation
- Lowered immune system strength
- Tumor growth
- More "rigid" cell walls and, therefore, altered cell function

Note: Many Omega-6s are linked to processed foods and also with meat intake, especially beef. Animals fed high grain diets (particularly in corn-fed beef), experience changes in their body chemistry, making the animal fats we consume "more inflammatory" than that of free-range animals (grass-fed beef).

The average American needs more Omega-3s, but we tend to eat more Omega-6s, which can cause an imbalance and send the body into an inflammatory state. Both Omega-3s and Omega-6s are important; just be sure to focus on increasing Omega-3s. This is what the balance should look like with the most common sources of the oils:

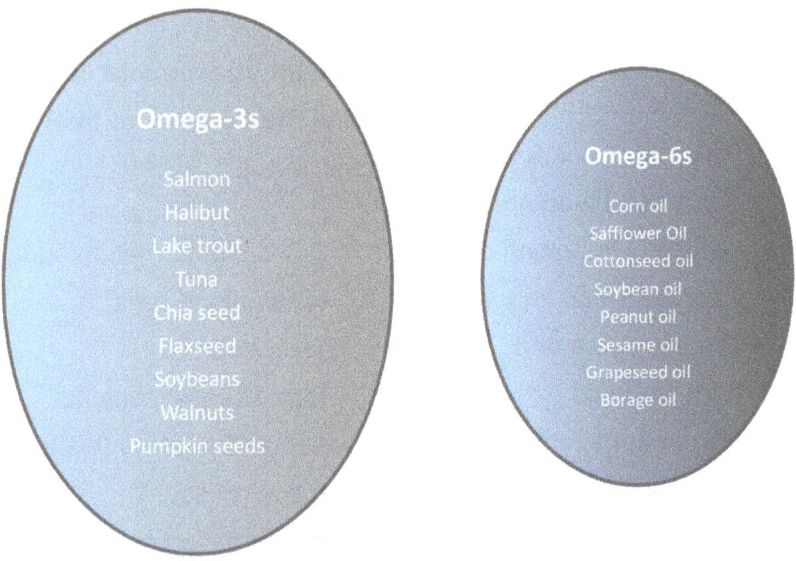

Rebalancing Omega-3s and Omega-6s

Saturated Fats—Saturated fats have been known for raising total blood-cholesterol levels, increasing low-density lipoproteins (LDLs - "bad cholesterol"), and increasing risk of heart disease when eaten in large amounts.

- Primary sources: **meat and dairy products, palm and coconut oils**

However, is this the full story? **Although saturated fats are traditionally labeled "bad," this may not entirely be the case.** Recent studies are showing saturated fats do not increase heart disease or stroke risk. Harvard Public Health reports on a review of studies over 23 years concluding, "There is insufficient evidence from prospective epidemiologic studies to conclude that dietary saturated fat is associated with an increased risk of CHD (coronary heart disease), stroke, or CVD (cardiovascular disease)."[61]

A summary of recent research in Progress in Cardiovascular Diseases states that refined sugars are a greater contributor to heart disease than saturated fats. In fact, some saturated fats actually have protective action and reduce the risk of heart disease, whereas the study found that high sugar consumption for just a few weeks changed the blood levels associated with heart disease risk factors, including high cholesterol, triglycerides, insulin resistance and abnormal glucose tolerance, low HDL, and more.[62]

Often, nutritional guidelines are greatly influenced and even determined by the food industry and other agencies that stand to profit from the "almighty dollar." The sugar industry was just one example of this exposure. In 2016, the *New York Times* reported that:

- In 1967, the Sugar Association paid off Harvard researchers to publish a research review based on the industry's hand-picked articles that **downplayed the association between sugar and heart disease, casting the blame instead on**

saturated fat and likely shaping much of the research on nutrition and heart disease.

- In 2015, Coca-Cola paid millions to downplay the link between sugary drinks and obesity.
- In 2016, candy makers' funds went toward reporting research that "children who eat candy tend to weigh less than those who do not."[63]

Some forms of saturated fats, **coconut oil** in particular, give us an entirely different story. Coconut oil has actually been called "one of the healthiest oils on earth." Cultures that traditionally use more coconut oil have lower rates of heart disease than those that don't. It's when these Eastern cultures become Westernized, adopting our cultural foods and diet, that their rates of heart disease increase.

Coconut oil has been used for generations around the world because of its reported wide range of health benefits and healing properties. Its unique molecular structure makes it easy to digest, converting it into energy and making it less likely to be stored as fat. Its high melting point makes it a great, stable choice for cooking. Use it lightly to prevent adding a coconut flavor, though much of the flavor will disappear with cooking and baking.

Coconut oil can work to:

- Increase metabolism and support thyroid function
- Reduce body weight
- Decrease cholesterol
- Regulate blood sugars
- Kill bacteria and viruses
- Lower inflammation
- Strengthen the immune system

The bottom line is that **we must carefully examine and discern what we've been taught.** Is the information true? Is it biased? What is it based on? It is safest to choose variety, moderation, and real, minimally processed whole foods, and select meat, eggs, and dairy products from grass-fed, free-range, and humanely treated animals. These will best fuel and protect your body, minimizing imbalances that come from additives, chemicals, hormones, and processed, empty-calorie foods.

Trans fats—Trans fats are **"bad" fats** otherwise known as **hydrogenated** and **partially hydrogenated oils**. They are made when fats and oils are changed from their liquid-oil state to a solid form in order to extend product shelf-life and to create a smooth texture. This chemical process changes the oil's structure, developing free radicals and changing natural oils into toxic fats. This not only destroys their health benefits but harms the body. These man-made fats:

- Are **associated with the highest risk of heart disease**
- Cause cells to become more "rigid" due to their new chemical structure
- Usually make up 5 to 10 percent of the standard American diet
- Are so unhealthy that a 1997 study in *New England Journal of Medicine* reports that **replacing just 2 percent** of trans-fat calories with non-hydrogenated, unsaturated fat, **will lower your risk of heart disease by 53 percent**
  - Primary sources: hydrogenated vegetable oils and partially hydrogenated oils, primarily found in **peanut butter, packaged crackers, cookies,**

snacks, bakery items, biscuits, doughnuts, fried foods, frosting, salad dressings, margarine, and shortening.

Trans fats are such a health risk that in June of 2015, the FDA began cracking down on their use in food production, allowing producers three years to come into compliance. These regulations allow companies to either reformulate items or petition for approval for use.[64] Label reading is important in order for you to know what items commonly use hydrogenated oils. A food label is permitted to list zero grams as long as it uses less than 0.5 grams of trans fats. However, this small amount can still add up over time; it only takes a relatively small amount of trans fats to have adverse effects.

Nuts—Nuts are mostly known for their **"good fats."** Each variety also contains antioxidants, vitamins, minerals, fiber, and protein. The nutrients in nuts work in synergy, giving incredible health benefits. Nuts can help your body:

- Lower blood pressure
- Raise HDLs (good cholesterol) and lower LDLs (bad cholesterol), reducing heart disease risks
  - In 2004, the FDA approved the first qualified health claim to be printed on packaging for walnuts, showing the relationship between nut intake and a **reduced risk of heart disease**.
  - Eating nuts four times each week showed a 37 percent reduction of heart disease compared with those who didn't eat nuts. Each additional serving reduced heart disease 8.3 percent and improved

blood vessel elasticity, and thus, blood vessel health, by 64 percent.[65]

- Promote improved brain function
- Reduce inflammation throughout the body
- Improve one's mood and reduce depression and behavioral disorders
- Reduce the risk of having a stroke[66] or developing type 2 diabetes,[67] dementia,[68] macular degeneration,[69] and gallstones[70]
- Help maintain healthy body weight
  - Frequent nut consumption is associated with a **reduced risk of weight gain**. People who ate nuts more than two times each week were 31 percent less likely to gain weight than those who did not.[71]
- Delicious choices include **almonds, walnuts, pecans, cashews, macadamia nuts, pistachios, and Brazil nuts**

A small handful of nuts fills you up and satisfies, discouraging empty-calorie snacking.

Spice It Up

Americans traditionally season food with salt and pepper. As a nation, we aren't typically familiar with the huge variety of herbs and spices available, nor do we know how to use them in the kitchen. However, most other **cultures use numerous herbs and spices, which go a long way in flavor balancing.**

Loaded with antioxidants and phytochemicals, the nutritional benefits of herbs are huge. As little as one gram of herbs per day can significantly raise antioxidant levels.

Research documents the benefits of herbs and spices. Here's just a short list of what herbs and spices can do: [72]

- Prevent and protect against cancer formation and growth
- Protect cells and DNA from free radicals and oxidation
- Regulate and lower blood sugars
- Give antiviral, antimicrobial, and antibacterial properties
- Reduce inflammation
- Alleviate stomach distress and nausea
- Improve circulation

Use the short guide below to start experimenting in your kitchen, opening up a new world of flavors and making your food more exciting—and nutrient dense! Dried (preferably organic) herbs work well, but most can be found fresh in the grocery produce section, and these can be frozen or dried for later use. Better yet, grow your own for use at any time.

Basil—Italian, Thai, Mediterranean, Indian dishes

Mix with tomatoes and tomato dishes, pesto, salads, Italian dishes, and stir-frys.

- Has antioxidant, anticancer, antibacterial, and antiviral benefits

Cinnamon—Asian, Middle Eastern, African

Use with apples, pears, sweet potatoes, pumpkin, cereals/grains, poultry, and vegetable stews.

- Has blood sugar regulator and strong antioxidant properties

Ginger—Asian, Indian dishes, Middle Eastern

Add to stir-frys, sauces, marinades, dressings, green smoothies, and sprinkle on sweet potatoes. To make ginger tea, grate or slice fresh ginger, steep with boiling water, and add a touch of honey.

- Is anti-inflammatory, a pain reliever, a potent cancer fighter, and a tummy calmer, alleviating GI distress and nausea (including motion and morning sickness)

Garlic—Italian, Asian, Thai, Mexican, Latin, Cajun, Indian, Middle Eastern dishes

Use in salads, stir-frys, dressings, sauces, and marinades for meats and veggie dishes, including greens, tomatoes, cucumbers, peppers, onions, avocados, and asparagus. Also blends well with many other herbs.

- Is anti-inflammatory, an immune booster, a cancer fighter, and a heart protector

Cilantro—Mexican, Indian, Asian dishes

Use in salsa, guacamole, eggs, salads, stir-frys, coconut curry, spring rolls, to garnish tacos, chili, lime chicken, and brown rice.

- Has antidiabetic and heavy-metal chelator properties

Mustard seed—French, Chinese, Indian dishes

Use for mustard, salad dressings, sauces, meat spreads or marinades, and stir-frys. Blends well with garlic, ginger, vinegar, and honey.

- Is a cancer fighter, anti-inflammatory, and a potent antioxidant

Parsley—Middle Eastern, French, Italian dishes

Use in Tabbouleh, soups, stews, salads, veggies, meat, fish, eggs, and pasta. Pairs well with mushrooms and tomatoes.

- Has strong antioxidant and cancer-fighting properties

Rosemary—Mediterranean dishes

Use in salad dressings, soups, eggs, meat, fish, poultry, bean stews, grains, and infused olive oils.

- Improves circulation and is anti-inflammatory, a strong antioxidant, and a cancer fighter

Turmeric—(the main spice in **curry**)—Indian, Asian, Middle Eastern dishes

Use with cauliflower, rice, veggies, lentils, garbanzo beans, eggs, chicken, greens, and fish. (Use caution, as turmeric stains easily.)

- Has powerful anti-inflammatory properties comparable to some medications, and has potent anticancer properties[73]

Sea salt

Contains essential trace minerals that have not been processed, added, or removed. Look for color (gray, pink) to identify extra minerals.

- Is a fluid and electrolyte balancer, affecting almost every cell and body process

Clearly, there is plenty you *can* eat! Our biggest challenge: we've gotten away from what many of the options are, how to prepare them, creatively plan with them and even blend flavors. Just think…it's a whole new food world waiting to be explored!

Here is the next key to making healthy delicious: **find real-food alternatives to your favorite processed, empty-calorie foods.** Your choices of real food are endless, a whole treasure chest just waiting to be discovered. Learning how to work with even a few new ingredients can open up a whole new world of dining experiences and favorites for you. And lest you fear that it's all veggies and savory flavors from here on out, let's see how to do healthy *starting with dessert.*

Be Revitalized

What are three things you will tweak in your eating to make sure you have a solid foundation and structure that will be delicious?

1.

2.

3.

How to Make Healthy Start with Dessert

We usually think that desserts are the first thing to go in a healthy lifestyle. But with a new perspective and a creative look at satisfying your sweet tooth, desserts can still fit right into your new lifestyle!

Naturally Sweet and Sugar-less

For those of you with a sweet tooth, this *does not* mean you'll never enjoy sweet indulgences again. Believe me! It just means you'll be **switching to new sources for sweets**. You'll be shocked to find that you enjoy their richer, deeper flavors even more than their empty-calorie counterparts.

Sugar, besides being loaded with empty calories (think soda) has some of the most detrimental effects on our body. As noted earlier, the average American eats an astronomical *142 pounds of processed sugars each year*. It's everywhere—salad dressings, soups, cereals, breads, desserts, crackers, and beverages of all types, even fruit juices! It's shocking to see the sugars add up. And here's the sneaky thing. Just check the label of any of your favorite foods. **Sugar goes by many, many names**. Here are just a few:

Barley malt syrup
Beet sugar
Brown rice syrup
Brown sugar
Cane crystals
Cane sugar
Corn sweetener
Corn syrup
Corn syrup solids
Dehydrated cane juice
Dextrin
Dextrose
Evaporated cane juice
Fructose
Fruit juice concentrate
Glucose
High-fructose corn syrup
Invert sugar
Maltodextrin
Malt syrup
Maltose
Molasses
Raw sugar
Rice syrup
Sorghum
Sorghum syrup
Sucrose
Syrup
Treacle
Turbinado sugar
Xylose

Certainly a little sugar now and then won't affect your health . . . right? Wrong. Did you know that **as little as one teaspoon of sugar can compromise your immune system for up to six hours**? Poor regulation of glucose and insulin levels produce free radicals (think browning apples again) in the body. This stimulates the body's inflammation response and taxes the immune system when continued over time. This may sound trivial, but recent research names chronic inflammation as one of the main contributing factors to most chronic, degenerative diseases and aging.[74] It is especially known as being the root cause of cancer and heart disease but high inflammatory markers are also found in many other conditions, including depression, allergies, arthritis, and psoriasis.

Here's a short list of some of the 146 research-documented **ways that sugar affects the body**, compiled by Nancy Appleton, PhD, in her book *Suicide by Sugar*:

- Suppresses the immune system
- Feeds cancer cells
- Is an addictive substance
- Depletes mineral levels, affecting bone health
- Causes tooth decay and periodontal disease
- Disrupts blood sugar and insulin levels, increasing the risk of diabetes
- Contributes to obesity
- Can cause hyperactivity, anxiety, and the inability to concentrate
- Worsens symptoms of ADHD
- Reduces learning capacity and plays a role in learning disorders
- Compromises GI health
- Affects digestion. Sugar is the number-one enemy of healthy bowel movements. It slows transit time, causes constipation, feeds Candida (yeast infections), and raises the risk of Crohn's disease, ulcerative colitis, and irritable bowel syndrome.
- Leads to hormonal imbalances
- Decreases tissue elasticity and function, and causes premature aging, especially for skin
- Can affect vision, causing nearsightedness, cataracts, and weakened eyesight

I encourage you to check out the complete list.[75]

One of the major impacts of sugar is seen in the GI tract. Over **70 percent of the immune system is linked to the gastrointestinal tract**, as it is home to a huge number of the immune system's cells and tissues.[76] High amounts of sugar and refined, processed foods can promote an overgrowth of unhealthy bacteria, yeast, and fungi. This throws off the "good bacteria" balance, which can result in less frequent bowel movements and toxin buildup, ultimately compromising the immune system, not to mention causing numerous unpleasant symptoms throughout the body. Studies are even beginning to address the possibility that this bacteria imbalance could be playing a unique role in our nation's obesity issues.

Sugar can also have a huge impact on the brain. Neurology research in Dr. Caroline Leaf's *Who Switched Off My Brain?* shows that sweets, along with refined pasta and breads, act as comfort foods, boosting brain serotonin and improving one's mood, at least for a short time. However, this mood boost lasts just twenty minutes. Neurologist David Perlmutter's extensive research on healthy lifestyles and brain health concludes that "**sugar and carbohydrates represent a powerful threat to the brain**." His review of a 2013 *Neurology* study shows the "dramatic" association between blood sugar levels and brain function and structure. Higher blood sugar levels were associated with the shrinking of the memory center of the brain (the hippocampus), while lower blood sugar levels were associated with better learning abilities and memory recall[77, 78] Think about what this means for kids of all ages.

Taking brain changes a step farther, some are now considering Alzheimer's disease to be "type 3 diabetes." The *Alzheimer's Society of Canada* explains that type 2 diabetes is a risk factor for Alzheimer's and dementia and is related to the associated cardiovascular issues (high blood pressure, high cholesterol, impaired circulation) and changes from high blood sugar levels. Furthermore, as with diabetes, the brains of Alzheimer's patients are unable to properly use glucose. Studies show that these patients' brains are in a "diabetic state," often due to insulin resistance and low insulin levels.[79]

As for sugar addictions, they are very real. In a 2009 ABC news story, Dr. Joe McClernon of Duke University discussed how the brain centers respond to high fat and high sugar foods similarly to how they respond to cocaine and smoking, especially in the brains of those struggling with obesity. Dr. Louis J. Aronne, a clinical professor at Weill Cornell Medical School and former president of the Obesity Society, puts it this way, "Your brain reacts almost identically to [that of] a cocaine addict looking at cocaine."[80]

Think **artificial sweeteners** are the way to go? Not so much! Those cute colored packets give more than just a few moments of sweet taste, filling your body with chemicals it doesn't know what to do with. A study published in the America Diabetes Association's 2009 *Diabetes Care Journal* reveals that diet sodas actually increased the risk of type 2 diabetes. Drinking diet sodas daily was associated with a **36 percent greater risk of metabolic syndrome** (a cluster of symptoms that increase your risk for diabetes and heart disease) and a **67 percent increased risk of type 2 diabetes** compared to no diet sodas.[81] Cleveland Clinic's Medical Director, Mark Hyman's review of a 2013 *American Journal of Clinical Nutrition* study also showed that diet sodas actually increased the risk of type 2 diabetes more than sugar-sweetened sodas. Women drinking one twelve-ounce diet soda weekly experienced a 33 percent increased risk of type 2 diabetes, while women drinking one twenty-ounce diet soda weekly had a 66 percent increased risk. That's twice as high, with just an extra eight ounces each week! Hyman summarizes this research, saying diet-soda drinkers run a **200 percent higher obesity risk**.[82,83,84, 85] Here are a few other facts on artificial sweeteners:

- Taste one hundred to one thousand times sweeter than regular sugar, activating our brains and taste buds to prefer sweets over other flavors[86]
- Trigger cravings for more sugar and starchy carbs
- Trick our metabolism into thinking sugar is coming, releasing insulin and triggering abdominal fat storage
- Confuse and slow our metabolism, causing us to burn fewer calories daily
- Alter the bacteria balance in the digestive tract, which can affect blood sugar regulation and increase weight gain[87]
- Increase belly fat
  - Diet soda drinkers gained nearly three times the abdominal fat in nine years compared to non-diet-soda drinkers, according to a 2015 article in the *Journal of the American Geriatrics Society*.[88]
- Add body fat
  - In animal studies, artificial sweeteners increased body fat by 14 percent in just two weeks, even with the test subjects eating fewer calories.
- Can cause side effects
  - More than sixty-eight studies document adverse effects from artificial sweeteners: behavioral and mood changes, convulsions and seizures, headaches, migraines, weight gain, and increased appetite.[89]

So what do you do with a sweet tooth, since sugar and artificial sweeteners so negatively affect the body? Check out the numerous natural sweeteners that can give you sweet pleasure while actually benefiting the body. Here are some options:

Natural Sweetener	**Health Benefits**
Raw Honey Very thick, usually creamy and opaque	– Strengthens the immune system – Can improve seasonal (and regional) allergies – Can improve blood sugars in type 2 diabetics – Antibacterial, antifungal, and antiviral properties – Rich in vitamins and minerals – High antioxidant content: comparable to fruits and vegetables and strong enough to raise blood levels[90]
Stevia Powder or liquid form, plain or flavored	– Is ~250 times sweeter than sugar – Calorie-free – Doesn't raise blood sugar levels – Made from plant leaves
Pure Maple Syrup	– Lower glycemic than sugar (54 vs 63)[91] – Rich in minerals (manganese, zinc) and riboflavin (vitamin B2)[92] – High antioxidant content (65), ranking among fruits and vegetables[93]

Fruit, Fruit Puree, and Dried Fruit
(Bananas, dates, raisins, mangos, applesauce)
	– Full of antioxidants, phytonutrients, vitamins, minerals, and fiber:
	  – Slow aging
	  – Protect cells from free-radical damage
	  – Strengthen the immune system

Coconut Sugar Light brown granules	– Low-glycemic sweetener – Full of vitamins, minerals, and amino acids (minimally processed)
Xylitol (Birch Sugar) or Erythritol White granules	– A sugar alcohol: a carb slowly and incompletely absorbed by the body, resulting in fewer calories and slower blood sugar rise, requiring little to no insulin – Very low glycemic score, which helps maintain blood sugar levels – Virtually calorie-free – Known to inhibit growth of bacteria and to prevent cavities

	– May cause digestive upset in large quantities (which usually improves with gradual introduction)
Raw Agave Nectar Syrup	– Considered low-glycemic (fructose is broken down differently than other sugars in the liver) – Quite controversial, with its high and imbalanced fructose content and minimal research – Some manufacturers mix it with other sugary syrups – Avoid or use rarely in small amounts with caution

Tips for Using Natural Sweeteners

- Combine sweeteners for more balanced flavors. This keeps your recipe from tasting too much like stevia or honey, or from having too strong of a fruit flavor.
- Reduce oven temperature by about 25° if using maple syrup or honey, as your baked goods will brown faster.
- Be sure to use organic, non-GMO xylitol or erythritol. Often, these are corn-based, and you don't want to introduce the complications of GMO corn.
- Exchange xylitol for sugar in recipes at about a one-to-one ratio. However, xylitol can cause GI upset in large amounts. Introduce it slowly, and the body will adjust. Alternatively, mix it with other natural sweeteners or try erythritol.
- Substitute erythritol at about a one-third-higher rate than sugar in recipes, or combine with other natural sweeteners.
- Adjust liquids. If using raw honey or maple syrup, you may need to reduce the total liquid of your recipe.

- Adjust volumes if using stevia. Since it is so much sweeter than sugar, much less is needed, which can alter your ratios of dry and liquid ingredients.
- Choose your favorite natural sweetener for specific uses. I love stevia in coffee and in smoothies when needed, but I prefer honey in tea. Some recipes work better with stevia (especially more bitter or pungent flavors like lemon), while dried fruit works better in others.
- If you've tried stevia and don't like it, try a new brand, a different form, or another blend. (Some natural sweeteners have additional ingredients to make them easier to use, while some are concentrated extracts.) Each has a slightly different flavor depending on how it's made, its state (liquid or solid), and the presence of added ingredients. Some really do taste better than others. (KAL® Pure Stevia Extract is currently my favorite powder for recipes and coffee. I prefer Trader Joe's® Organic Liquid Stevia for iced tea, and SweetLeaf Stevia® for flavored liquid varieties.) Also, read labels carefully, as all stevias are not created equal, which affects quantities needed for sweetening.

My love of sweets, my first-hand knowledge of sugar's effects on the body, and my struggle with feeling deprived and dissatisfied from all the "—free" diets, led me to experimenting in the kitchen. My passion grew to inspire others to deliciously healthful, radiant living…starting with dessert! From a combination of nuts, fruits, favorite flavors and natural sweeteners, the Innocent Indulgence® raw dessert line was born, offering rich, creamy cheesecakes and moist, chewy cookie bars that actually nourish the body! As a family-owned business, Innocent Indulgence® produced and shipped desserts nationwide, supplying Arizona Whole Foods Markets®, New Frontier's Markets, and a variety of other local restaurants and special events for five years.

Innocent Indulgence's® former dessert line has proven how healthy *really can start* with and include sweet-tooth treats. By **uniquely combining, thinking creatively, and preparing ingredients differently**, the deliciousness you can enjoy is truly amazing! Check the recipe section at the end of the book for some incredibly yummy ideas and a selection of our favorite, signature desserts. Now you can make them in your own home. You won't be deprived. Moderation is still important, but by reducing and avoiding processed sweeteners, your body will enjoy *much* better health, and you can have "**all of the yum and none of the guilt**."

Here are some ideas to jumpstart your creativity for quick, sweet-snacking treats that you (and the kids) will love! You'll never miss the sugar…and your body will love you for it.

- Blend fruit smoothies: fruit, unsweetened milk alternative, ice, and raw honey or stevia to taste
  - Strawberry and banana
  - Orange, pineapple, banana, and coconut
  - Raspberries and mango
  - Cherries and cocoa protein powder
- Freeze fruit kabobs: alternate a variety of fruit chunks on a skewer
- Treat yourself to banana pops or a banana split
  - Cut bananas into 1-inch bites and load onto sticks

  - Coat with any combination of chopped nuts, coconut, cinnamon, cocoa, dried fruit, mini dark chocolate chips
  - Freeze pops OR
  - Cut banana lengthwise, place halves in a bowl, and load with favorite toppings (above)
- Make pecan pies: stuff dates with pecans and sprinkle with cinnamon
- Dip apple or banana slices in nut butter and sprinkle with cinnamon and raisins
- Revise your favorite holiday recipes and replace sugars with natural sweeteners
- Whip up no-bake cookies with nut butters, cocoa or dark chocolate chunks, dried fruit, pumpkin seeds, oats, spices and raw honey
- Sip an assortment of sparkling waters or unsweet teas
  - Garnish with a slice of fruit or berries (sweeten with stevia or a touch of honey if desired)
  - Try Zevia® (a stevia-sweetened soda) instead of sugary sodas

Now, let's get you set up to succeed on your new lifestyle with some meal guidelines to get you moving forward on your journey.

Be Revitalized

What new ideas will you try to better satisfy your sweet tooth?

1.

2.

3.

4.

5.

What new sweet treats will you keep stocked to nip sugar indulgences?

1.

2.

3.

5

How to Make Healthy Daily

Making something new a part of your daily lifestyle isn't necessarily hard, it's just, well . . . *different*! At first, it will require more planning, changes of routine, a fresh way of operating, new plans, new recipes, new grocery lists, new stores, new choices, and more effort. It just plain takes time and repetition to establish a new normal. So, let's get started with some plans that will make this work for you.

What to Eat

You've probably seen the food guide pyramid before. It was modified a few years ago to MyPlate by the US Department of Agriculture Center for Nutrition Policy and Promotion. Here's my version, developed from my professional and personal experiences. It helps by giving a **visual of daily variety, how to balance foods and meals**, and it forms a more complete picture of health and wellness, showing where the focus should be. Let's start with the basics.

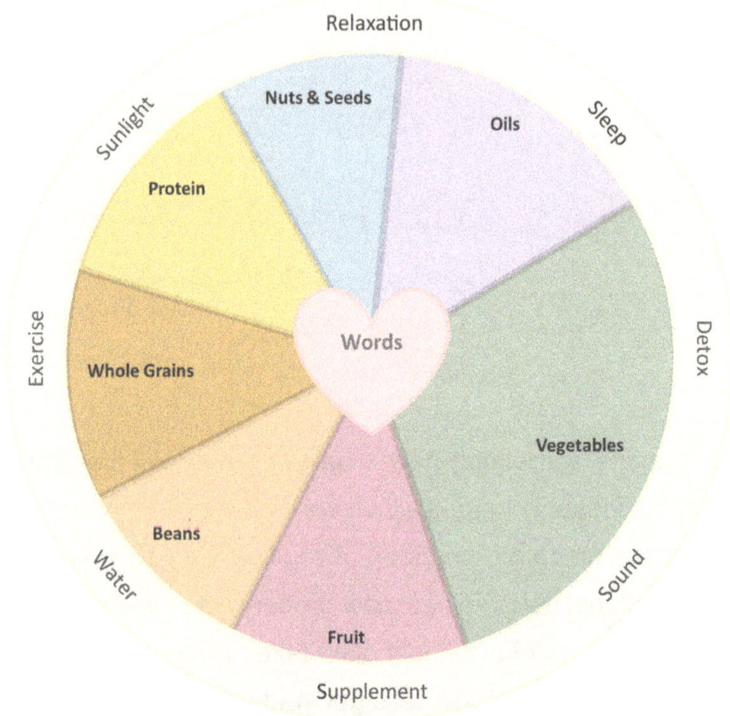

Whole Body Nutrition

The Plan

As you can see, the **majority of our food should come from plant sources: vegetables, fruit, nuts, beans, seeds, and whole grains, complemented with lean forms of protein**. Please note, with the exception of fruit and veggies, the number of recommended servings may vary, based on personal goals: needed weight loss, gain, or maintenance, healing, pregnancy, etc.However, the recommend portions below are an excellent starting point.

Vegetables—Four to six (4-6) servings minimum

Sound scary? It's not—and it's possible. Here's how:

	SERVING	LOOKS LIKE
Chopped vegetables – cooked	½ cup	half a baseball
Chopped vegetables – raw	1 cup	a baseball
Leafy greens	1 cup	a baseball OR a handful

Eat a salad every day, and think "salad bar" when building it. The more vegetables, the better!

Salads

Here's an example:

Base greens: romaine or spinach

Toppings: tomatoes, cucumbers, carrots, onions, and peppers

3 handfuls greens (3 servings) + ¼ cup x 4 veggies (1 serving) = 4 servings total

So, with just one simple salad, and without eating any other veggies during the day, you can easily reach four servings of vegetables.

Lettuce wraps

Need a break from salads? Try lettuce wraps. It's amazing what you can stuff into a lettuce leaf. Even more incredible, it seems you're eating an entirely different entrée. Load butter leaf, romaine, cabbage, chard, or kale (stiffer leaves roll and hold better) with a variety of veggies, beans, lean protein, sprouts, and avocado, and top with any sauce you love: dressing, hummus, spicy mustard, pesto, salsa, or sun-dried tomato spread.

Green smoothies

Drinking veggies is often quicker and more preferable than eating them, and the full nutrient content, **including fiber**, is preserved in the process. If you're new to green smoothies, start with spinach (which is slightly sweet) or romaine. Their mild taste makes for an easier adjustment. Also, start with a few leaves or just a handful, then work your way up as your taste buds get recalibrated.

> 3 handfuls of dark greens (3 servings) + 1-2 fruit servings = 4-5 servings total

Adding your favorite fruit, flavors, or other natural sweeteners can mask the bitter flavor of the greens, while ice, water, or almond milk can help thin the consistency. I personally love adding pear, pineapple, lime, banana, and ginger (mint works too) to offset the "green" flavor (See recipe section.)

Keys to a tasty green smoothie:

- A high-powered blender—Without it, you will end up with a chunky, gritty "smoothie," which can be a challenge for anyone, especially those who have "texture issues."
- Fruit—Fruit masks the strong green flavor. Bananas, mangos, limes or lemons, grapefruit, oranges, pineapple,

pears, and apples are among the best, and will keep your smoothie green rather than turning it brown.

  - Berries provide fabulous nutritional benefits, but be prepared for them to turn the smoothie a muddy-brown color.

- Stevia—This natural sweetener helps offset the bitter greens. Just be cautious to avoid over-sweetening, which can cause a strong bittersweet flavor. If you are at a juice bar, you might ask for their ingredient list or tell them to hold the sweeteners, as these drinks can often be loaded with surprise sugars, syrup-sweetened fruit, or a fruit juice base.
- Ice and liquid—Add enough ice and liquid to fit your preferences for an icy, thick, or thin smoothie. Everyone is different, but including ice and liquid is key to smooth blending.

Juicing

Fresh vegetable juices should really be a supplement, not a replacement for whole veggies. Juicing extracts and removes fiber, allowing for easy, quick absorption of the juice's freshly squeezed nutrients. The volume of produce required to make juice is truly unrivaled compared with what could possibly be eaten, and it allows for an **immediate infusion of nutrition**.

For example, if you were to make orange juice, you'd need to use at least three to four oranges to get one glass. Most people don't sit down and eat three to four oranges at once. Just think of the amount of spinach leaves required to make a glass of juice! Again, that quantity is much more than you would choose to eat in one sitting. But, oh, the nutrient density and quantity of vitamins, minerals, antioxidants, and phytonutrients in that concentrated drink!

The benefits of juicing (and testimonies of juicers) are truly incredible, but juicing is time-consuming, and is not the right starting place for everyone. If you choose to juice, I recommend making vegetable-based juices, using only moderate amounts of fruit for flavor balancing. (Skip ahead to see fruit juice notes in the Fruit section below.)

Seven servings of potatoes don't count

Note that the nutrient content of starchy veggies is just not quite the same as leafy greens. Carrots, beets, sweet potatoes, potatoes, and other varieties of winter squash have great benefits and are a good source of carbs (quick energy), but these should be kept to one or two of your five to seven daily servings.

Endless vegetable options:

- Stir-frys
- Steamed veggies can substitute for (or reduce) pasta
- Soups or stews loaded with veggies
- Veggies and dips
- Veggies added to sandwiches, wraps, burritos, and eggs
- Baked veggie meal combos or casseroles
- Blender soups, both hot and cold
- Pick your favorite sides: steamed, stir-fried, grilled or baked

Fruit—Two to four (2-4) servings

	Serving	Looks Like
Fresh	1 medium piece	a baseball
	1 cup chopped	a baseball
	1½ cups berries	a handful
Dried	¼ cup	a golf ball

Smoothies

Making this goal is not scary (or impossible) with **a smoothie a day**! Combine fruit blends with nondairy milks, a little water, or ice, and add a touch of stevia or honey if needed. Add a few greens if you'd like, or you can choose a 100 percent fruit smoothie. Either option is a great way to get two to three fruit servings.

Skip fruit juice

Remember, juicing removes the fiber and provides an unnatural number of fruit servings in a single sitting. Think of the number of oranges that go into a glass of juice (three or four); this gives you a straight shot of natural sugars that raises blood sugar levels higher and quicker.

Fresh fruit

Prefer to eat it instead of drink it? Try this:

- Sprinkle fresh berries on oatmeal or other grains
- Spread apple or banana slices with nut butter
- Slice melons, oranges, or other favorites for a quick snack or "dessert"
- Give salads a delicious flavor burst with fresh or dried fruit

- Blend frozen fruit with a touch of ice or milk as an alternative to gelato or ice cream
- Explore the possibilities

Just by making these additions, without any other changes (or eliminations), I can just about guarantee that you'll see some sort of improvement in health. These tips are foundational.

Beans—One to three (1-3) servings

	SERVING	LOOKS LIKE
Black, great northern, cannellini, garbanzo, lentils, kidney, pinto, white, navy, black-eyed peas, split peas	½ cup cooked	half a baseball

Beans are an **excellent source of protein and fiber**, which is important since most Americans need more to reach the *daily recommended* **thirty to forty grams of fiber**. "Regularity" is essential to keeping the "garbage" going out, preventing buildup in the colon, and stopping toxins from being reabsorbed back into your body. Here are some ways to eat more beans:

- Add to salads
- Toss in soups
- Roll up in wraps
- Use as a base and topped with chopped veggies, herbs, avocado, or grated cheese
- Puree into hummus or other bean dips for veggies, crackers, and other flavorful spreads
- Serve as a side dish

To make them more easily digestible, rinse beans well (especially if using canned varieties).

Whole Grains—One to three (1-3) servings

	Serving	Looks Like
Rice, cereal, pasta	½ cup	half a baseball
Amaranth, buckwheat, millet, quinoa, teff, organic corn, oatmeal	~½ cup	half a baseball
Whole-grain bread	1 slice	1 slice
Tortillas or pitas (large)	½	half a Frisbee

We do need some carbs for energy. Typically, the majority of grains are consumed as highly-processed "fluffy" calories. Processing removes much of their fiber, vitamins, minerals, and other antioxidants and phytonutrients. Thus, it's important to focus on whole grains. Read labels or buy and prepare grains in their basic form. Branch out and try lesser-known grains. Let your creativity kick in. You'll be amazed! Look for at least three grams of fiber in each serving.

What about gluten-free?

"Gluten-free" has become one of the latest food fads. But what is gluten, and why all the talk about it? First of all, gluten is a protein found most commonly in wheat, rye, barley, any other wheat varieties and products, and any food containing these ingredients. Partly, the awareness of the effects of gluten has risen as celiac rates have risen drastically in the last few years, with one out of 133 being diagnosed with the condition.[94] Here are a few terms you should know, as you'll see them often associated with gluten-free.

- **Celiac disease**—An autoimmune disease causing inflammation when wheat is consumed, triggering the body to attack and eat away at the lining of the small intestine. This impairs the body from properly digesting and absorbing foods, quite often leading to nutrient deficiencies and a host of other related conditions.
- **Non-celiac gluten sensitivity**—A term coined by experts in 2011 for someone who doesn't have true celiac disease, but who experiences better health and reduction of negative symptoms (e.g., skin, digestive) when not eating gluten, and whose health declines when gluten is reintroduced.
- **Food allergies**—There are two common types of food allergies:
  - Immediate (IgE) – The body's immune system produces antibodies to the food. Reactions are typically immediate (a few minutes to a couple of hours), and often have severe effects on breathing, skin, digestion, and even the heart.
  - Delayed (IgG or IgA) – These allergic reactions do not involve the immune system in the same way. Reactions typically are less severe and may even be delayed up to three to five days. Symptoms may include headaches, skin conditions, digestive issues, hormone imbalances, and foggy thinking.

So, what caused the change of public opinion about wheat? No one is certain, and the topic has become quite controversial, potentially because the incidence of testing for Celiac and food allergies has increased, while at the same time a true surge in wheat intolerance has emerged. **Or is it that the wheat itself has changed?**

To make wheat resistant to environmental changes (e.g., drought, fungus) and to increase harvest and crop yields, it has been hybridized and crossbred, drastically changing the genetic code of the plants' proteins. One of the earliest varieties of wheat studied had only fourteen chromosomes, while the wheat we eat today has been naturally and unnaturally crossed to contain forty-two chromosomes, making it **very complex genetically and hardly the same plant**. In fact, the new stalks are dwarfed varieties at one to two feet tall (hardly "amber waves of grain") and would struggle to survive without specialized, compatible fertilizer and pest control.[95] Here are a couple more of the changes:

- Lowered protein levels with a different carbohydrate composition that is high in **amylopectin-A**. This unique carb is **easily digested and rapidly converted to glucose, raising blood sugars higher than almost any other food**. Research shows the Glycemic Index, GI, (a measurement comparing types of carbohydrates' effects on blood sugar levels) of wheat bread is seventy-two, which is actually higher than GI of table sugar: fifty-nine.[96] This rise can easily contribute to weight gain and inflammation throughout the body.[97]
- Altered structure of **gliadin protein**, the second primary protein in wheat, which was nearly absent from wheat prior to the 1960s. This has been associated with triggering the intestinal changes occurring with celiac disease.[98] Modified gliadin proteins can also have a **"morphine like effect"**

and stimulate appetite. One study reported individuals consuming more than 400 extra calories per day.[99]

- Modified structure of **wheat germ agglutinin** (part of gliadin), which has a direct **damaging effect on the small intestine**. In addition, it may **block leptin**, a satiety (feeling full) hormone, contributing to weight gain.

Curiously enough, **gluten sensitivity may not have anything to do with the gluten**, but actually with the gliadin. And what about the fact that many gluten-containing foods are also foods that are typically high in an unnatural, highly processed form of wheat that has been, refined, and bleached, in addition to being treated with numerous pesticides, hormones, fungicides, and insecticides? Could the digestive symptoms, allergic-type reactions and other seemingly unexplained symptoms attributed to gluten actually be from the processed foods' lack of nutrients and the abundance of foreign chemicals they introduce into the body?[100] It will be fascinating to watch the research and information continue to emerge on this topic.

In addition to the more common digestive symptoms, in his book, *Wheat Belly,* Dr. William Davis sites numerous studies documenting that **wheat can affect the body from head to toe** in the following ways:

- Weight gain (especially fat deposits around organs)
- Insulin resistance and diabetes
- Elevated triglycerides and cholesterol levels
- Outbursts in those with ADHD and autism
- Coordination and balance issues, stemming from impacts on the brain

- More erratic behavior from people with schizophrenia
- Mood changes
- Migraines
- Lower energy
- Poor sleep
- Hair loss
- Aging effects on skin
- Acne
- Rashes on elbows and knees
- Accelerated aging process as a result of high blood sugar levels damaging cells in the blood vessels: eyes, heart, brain, and kidneys[101]

To eat wheat or not to eat wheat?

Although the developing body of research on gluten sensitivity, digestive concerns, and wheat-related reactions/issues may not be fully conclusive, many people really do feel better by removing wheat and/or gluten from their daily menus. Professionally, I want to get someone feeling better first with symptom management, which often can be *greatly improved* through food(s) and nutrition by removing potential allergenic or inflammatory items. Then, we can address deeper underlying root issues that usually take longer to nourish and rebalance. I suggest that many do at least a trial of gluten-free eating, or in other words, detox from highly-processed wheat products. Doing a **gluten-free trial** is a great starting point **especially if you experience digestive difficulties, battle with your weight, struggle to control your blood sugars as a diabetic, experience moods swings or behavioral disorders, or**

suffer with skin conditions such as eczema, acne, psoriasis, or hives.

It may take *four to six weeks* to completely flush wheat from your system, so you'll want to be strict during this time to have an accurate trial, especially if you're highly sensitive. You may notice a difference right away, or it may be a gradual change before you feel better and realize some symptoms are gone.

Initially, it will likely take more time to shop and meal plan, but it will be worth it. Keep in mind that you may have withdrawal symptoms, almost like a wheat hangover. Wheat can truly be addictive, so give the symptoms time to clear. Once you have your initial symptoms managed, you can more comfortably pursue healing your gut and immune system and rebalancing your body for even better health.

Note: gluten-free doesn't necessarily mean healthy. Many, if not the majority, of gluten-free items have simply replaced wheat with other highly-processed ingredients (e.g., potato starch, tapioca starch, white rice), which lack fiber and nutrients, and are typically high glycemic (causing a rapid rise and fall in blood sugar levels). This can easily contribute to weight gain, and cause an inflammatory effect. When selecting gluten-free items, it's important to choose ones that are high fiber and minimally processed, and that do not contain large amounts of sugar. Keep to simple, more basic whole foods, and add lots of flavor with herbs, spices, and other real-food ingredients.

In general, I'm not anti-wheat, but I'm skeptical about what has been done to wheat that appears to benefit the agricultural and food industries, at the apparent expense of consumers. An organic, whole-grain wheat product that is fresh, unprocessed, and not chemically treated would be a better option than a processed wheat product. And, depending on *your* body, wheat and/or gluten can be reintroduced and tolerated occasionally with rebalancing, detoxing, and healing (with the exception of Celiac disease).

Ideally, Einkorn wheat (the original wheat) is the best choice if you choose to eat wheat regularly. It's non-hybridized, has the most nutrients, is well tolerated even by those who are gluten sensitive (with the same exception for Celiacs), and is not associated with the long list of side effects like traditional wheat. I've seen some amazing results and health improvements in those who have switched, especially in better digestive health and breakthroughs in weight plateaus.

So, what in the world do you eat if you choose a gluten-light or gluten-free lifestyle? There are plenty of other carb sources, and the food industry now offers many gluten-free alternatives to the items you can't live without. Again, the key is finding new, delicious alternatives, getting in your daily vegetable and fruit servings, and choosing minimally processed food when possible.

Here are a few of my favorite alternatives:

- **Flours and grains**—Buckwheat, millet, amaranth, quinoa, rice (wild, brown), bean flours (chickpea, garbanzo/fava), flaxseed meal, chia seed meal, coconut flour, nut meals (almond, walnut, pecan), gluten-free oats
- **Beans**—Black, kidney, garbanzo, pinto, refried, white, navy; hummus
- **Tortillas**—Tortillas made from non-GMO corn (I find rice tortillas to be like cardboard.)

- **Tamari or coconut aminos**—Soy sauce is actually made from wheat, so be sure to use one of the wheat-free (and low-sodium) varieties.
- **Veggies and squashes**—
  - Zucchini, summer squash, spaghetti squash, cauliflower, and portabella mushrooms make great pasta replacements and even base ingredient for pizza "crust"
  - Sweet potatoes, yams, butternut and acorn squash, potatoes and other starchy vegetables make great carb replacements
  - Greens (butter leaf, romaine, chard, cabbage, etc.) make great sandwich wraps
  - Tomatoes, cucumbers, peppers, zucchini, and mushrooms make great holders for protein salads, dips or guacamole (stuffed peppers, stuffed zucchini, tuna boats, etc.)

Nuts and Seeds—One to three (1-3) servings

	SERVING	LOOKS LIKE
Almonds, Brazil, cashews, hazelnuts, pecans, pine nuts, macadamia, pistachios, peanuts, walnuts; hemp, sesame, pumpkin, sunflower seeds	⅓ cup	a handful
Nut butter	2 tablespoons	half a golf ball

Selection is key. When possible, **choose raw or sprouted nuts**. Nuts are really a form of seed that, when planted, can grow and produce many more. "Life is in the seed." So, when they are soaked and sprouted to begin the life-giving process, the proteins break down into easily absorbed amino acids, increasing the protein content and making them easier to digest. Many roasted nut varieties add extra oils, refined salt and sugars, and then roast the nuts at high temperatures, which change their oil composition into forms that lower the benefits and even become harmful to the body. Instead, look for **nut butters seasoned with sea salt, without hydrogenated oils and added sugars**.

Move out of your usual nut rut; **try a few different kinds to give your body a variety of nutrients and additional health benefits**. Almonds have an alkalizing effect on the body, walnuts provide omega-3s, Brazil nuts supply selenium for thyroid and antioxidant support, and pumpkin seeds are high in zinc. Try small amounts from bulk nut bins, or look for small packages to help you taste test and find your new favorites.

Oils—Two to three (2-3) servings minimum

	Use	Form	Amount for Supplement Use*
Coconut Oil	– Baking, cooking and stir-frys – Supplement – High smoke point makes it a top choice for cooking	– Extra virgin, cold-pressed, expeller-pressed – Steam-deodorized is OK if you don't like the coconut flavor	1–3 tablespoons
Olive Oil	– Salads, dressings – Cooking (high quality EVOO has a high smoke point) – Quick cooking is ok; raw oil provides most benefits	– Extra virgin, cold pressed (EVOO)	1–3 tablespoons
Flaxseed Oil	– Omega-3 supplement – Salad dressings—combine oils for milder flavor – Smoothies – (Do not heat)	– Cold pressed – Keep refrigerated – (High-lignin oil has a very strong flavor)	1–2 tablespoons
Flaxseed**	– Egg or flour substitute – Fiber supplement (omega-3 benefits)	– Brown or golden seeds, ground	1–2 tablespoons
Chia Seed**	– Fiber supplement (omega-3 benefits)	– Seeds	1–4 tablespoons
Olives	– Condiment – Snack	– Kalamata, green, black, Spanish	5 small
Avocado	– Condiment – Snack – Avocado oil's high smoke point makes it a top choice for cooking	– Fresh – Cold pressed oil	¼–½ medium

*Based on health conditions, symptoms, and goals for weight gain or loss
**Add to smoothies, oatmeal, applesauce, or pumpkin with cinnamon; use instead of poppy seeds; or make chia seed pudding (almond or coconut milk and sweetener or flavored stevia drops—toffee, coffee, and/or vanilla)

Prepared salad dressings typically have high amounts of processed oils and low amounts of healthful oils, and use other less-than-desirable ingredients. Be sure to read labels and use sparingly, preferably making your own simple versions with olive oil, vinegar or citrus juice (i.e., lemon, lime, orange), and herbs, spices, and/or garlic.

Butter is fine. Choose organic when possible, as its fat structure is very important to cell health, especially in the GI tract. Avoid margarine, since it is loaded with trans fats.

Protein

	Serving	Looks Like
Red meat, poultry, fish	3 oz. (boneless, cooked weight from 4 oz. raw)	a deck of cards
Cheese	1½ oz.	4 die, or 2 nine-volt batteries
Egg	1 oz.	1 egg

Protein has become quite the controversial subject in the nutrition field, with recommendations ranging from high "overload" amounts to minimal amounts or totally avoiding sources of animal protein altogether. My brief recommendation is this: *it depends*.

Although I promote a **plant-rich, whole-foods lifestyle**, **protein needs really do vary.** Pregnancy, growth, weight loss, and healing from certain conditions require more protein. On the other hand, at least a short period of detoxing with animal-free, dairy-free eating is a good idea, especially for some serious health conditions. Really, *everyone* can benefit from short times of rest from animal proteins, which allow the body to cleanse itself of the toxins and chemicals that typically come along with these foods.

Since we digest and incorporate into our bodies the animals' diets and their medical treatments, it's important when eating meat and dairy to keep it as a condiment or a side rather than the focal point of the meal. Also, be sure to make **"clean" protein choices**:

- Organic
- Antibiotic-free
- Hormone-free
- Grass-fed
- Free-range
- Cage-free
- Wild fish
- Lean selections
- Avoid shellfish: lobster, crab, shrimp, oysters, clams, all farmed fish, and catfish

Make a mental switch and **start planning your meals around your veggie dishes** to keep your daily eating plant-rich. **Good sources of lean protein can be added to any veggie recipe or dish**, with the following ideas:

- Salads, wraps, or greens
- Veggie stir-fry blends
- Soups and stews
- Whole grain rice
- Bean dishes

I eat meat, eggs, and fish. I don't drink cow's milk by the glass, but I do like cheese and unsweetened yogurt (which I flavor with fruit and stevia), and I occasionally rotate in goat varieties. One of the biggest issues I've seen with going vegetarian or vegan is not getting enough protein. This can translate into a number of concerns: weakened immunity, blood sugar and hormone imbalances, muscle loss, difficulty concentrating, mood swings, slow wound healing, hair loss and weak nails. Ladies, healthy skin, hair, and nails require protein, and most of us want to maintain (and build) muscle, so protein is not something to skimp on. In general, include a good protein source at each meal.

Dairy

I recommend **keeping your dairy consumption light**. Stick with organic cheeses, yogurt, or kefir, since most of the milk sugars have been digested by the fermenting cultures and enzymes, minimizing GI upset. Plus, your body benefits from their strains of beneficial bacteria, boosting GI and immune system health. Organic gives a higher quality product with more important fatty acids and reduces the chemicals, growth hormones, antibiotics and pesticides typically found in conventional dairy. Typically, goat or sheep dairy is easier to digest than cow's milk and is not as "acidic" for the body. Keep in mind that dairy products rank high on the list of the top eight allergenic foods by the FDA, and overall, are quite a controversial topic in the field of nutrition.[102]

Soy

Soy is also controversial among nutritionists. I recommend **avoiding it**, or using organic (non-GMO) soy products only occasionally. I work with many individuals with digestive issues, and soy is one of the most common food allergies known for causing GI distress. Furthermore, soy-consuming cultures typically use fermented forms of soy, not the varieties of westernized soy products on our grocery shelves.

What to Drink

These recommendations are based strictly on hydration and nutrient density.

Water

Water is **essential to life**! We can live days and even weeks without food, yet only a few days without water. It's the basic element for all of life. Water makes up 75 percent of our entire body, but it is concentrated in some areas: the brain is 85 percent water, muscles are 75 percent water, bone is 22 percent water, and fat is 10 percent water. Water helps keep your entire body healthy and hydrated, **transporting nutrients into cells and clearing toxins out of cells and tissues**. Water works in our bodies in many ways:

- Biochemical reactions—Water keeps the body functioning and transports substances into, out of, and in-between cells.
- Blood—Water delivers oxygen and nutrients to the cells.
- Lymphatic system—Water carries away waste products and germs.
- Digestion—Water makes up saliva and digestive enzymes in the stomach, pancreas, and liver.
- Urine—Water excretes waste.
- Spinal fluid—Water allows for nerve transmission.
- Fluids—Water lubricates around the heart, lungs, abdominal organs, joints, and spinal column.
- Perspiration—Water helps regulate body temperature.
- Tears—Water cleanses the eyes.
- Mucus—Water protects from germs in the lungs, nose, and throat.
- Shock absorption—Water protects the spinal column and joints.
- Reproduction—Water supports fertility and hormone balances, and assists women in developing their babies during pregnancy and while breastfeeding.

We lose about nine to twelve cups of water naturally throughout the day without even exercising. This occurs through sweat, breathing, tears, feces, and urine. More water is also lost because of caffeine's diuretic effects via coffee, tea, and soft drinks. **When water losses are greater than water intake, dehydration occurs, moving water from inside to outside the cells in an attempt to rebalance the body's fluids. This fluid shift changes the cells' structures and, thus, their function, affecting every organ in the body.** Think of a plump, juicy grape versus a shriveled raisin. You want your cells like grapes, not raisins, for a healthy body and for organs, systems, and tissues to function properly.

Dehydration can cause the body to experience the following effects:

- Free-radical damage
- More rapid aging
- Damage to cell structure and tissues
- Waste-product build up
- Development of many disease states, including cancer, diabetes, autoimmune diseases, allergies, lupus, and asthma
- Worsening of symptoms, illnesses, and diseases
- Increase in blood pressure, inflammation, and blood clotting

Dehydration actually causes the same stress response in the body as an emotional stressor, since the brain cells must work to maintain their fluid balance. As little as a 3 percent loss of body water results in fatigue and organ dysfunction. At 4 percent loss, muscle strength and endurance drop, and a 10 percent loss in body water is life threatening. Usually thirst kicks in at about 1 to 2 percent loss of body water, but infants, the elderly, athletes, and those with illnesses often have unreliable thirst mechanisms and need to be encouraged to drink more fluids. Interestingly, long airline flights can cause the loss of up to six cups of fluid within three hours due to the dehumidified air in the plane. Be sure to drink extra fluids when traveling.

To calculate your daily fluid needs, **divide your body weight in half**. This gives you the **ounces of fluid you need to consume daily**. Be sure to factor in extra fluids for heat, humidity, travel, activity, and caffeine consumption.

Do you find yourself bored by plain water? Add a few drops of flavored stevia (which comes in an almost endless variety of flavors) to make water more exciting. Or add a splash of citrus with lemon, lime, or orange; frozen fruit like blackberries or raspberries; or even a cucumber slice to liven up your glass.

Coffee

I must mention coffee for all my fellow coffee-lovers. It's **rich in antioxidants and has many psychological and social benefits**. The *Scientific Report of the 2015 Dietary Guidelines Advisory Committee* from the Office of Disease Prevention and Health Promotion summarizes a significant amount of research on the connections between coffee and chronic disease. Its investigation shows **moderate coffee intake can lower the risks** of the following conditions:

- Type 2 diabetes
- Cardiovascular disease
- Liver cancer
- Alzheimer's disease & Parkinson's disease
- Cognitive decline (memory and thinking skills)[103]

It's best to choose organic beans and avoid the extra sugar, syrups, creamers, and dairy. I choose to keep my coffee consumption to one to two cups per day. I also make my own specialty coffee drinks with unsweetened coconut and almond milk that is warmed and frothed. I sweeten with stevia and sometimes add cinnamon, cocoa powder or pumpkin pie spice.

For those facing high levels of stress and adrenal fatigue, you might consider decaffeinating, at least for a time. Caffeine can continue to stress the adrenals, affecting the overall functioning of this very important gland: lowering energy, causing lethargy and muscle weakness, inability to deal with stress, blood sugar imbalances, hormone imbalances, increased allergic reactions, and a host of other symptoms in the long-run. Swiss Water® will give you the cleanest, no-chemical decaf coffee that still tastes terrific.

Tea: green, red (rooibos), black, white, herbal, oolong

Just pick your color and pour a cup! Sipping tea provides a host of benefits to the body, primarily through their **high antioxidant contents**. The colors and types simply describe their harvesting and "processing." Here's a crash course on the differences between teas and just a few of their many, many benefits:

	DESCRIPTION	BENEFITS
White tea	A pure form of tea that is the least processed with higher antioxidant contents, giving it a very delicate flavor	– Detoxifies the body – Fights cancer – Promotes weight loss – Improves and protects heart health
Green tea	Slightly oxidized during production, but is unfermented: – Japanese green tea is steamed – Chinese green tea is pan seared Green tea is probably the most widely researched tea	– Improves heart and artery health and lowers cholesterol – Reduces cancer risks and can block cancer-cell growth – Aids in weight loss, increases metabolism, and blocks fat absorption – Increases bone density and oral health – Has anti-inflammatory and anti-aging properties by helping to protect DNA – Can improve brain function and mental clarity
Oolong tea	Slightly more oxidized than green, and is partially fermented – Typically a Chinese tea	– Supports weight loss – Relieves eczema – Strengthens heart health and reduces blood pressure – Stabilizes blood sugar levels and diabetes – Relieves physical and mental stress
Black tea	Fully fermented – Think of sweet tea in the South	– Can improve heart health by increasing artery elasticity and reducing blood pressure
Herbal tea	Not an actual "tea," but is made by combining dried fruits, herbs, and flowers	– Relaxes and soothes the body – Often blended for therapeutic purposes
Red tea, or Rooibos	Made from the South African "red bush" Not a true "tea"	– Traditionally used to boost immune system and reduce allergy, asthma, and digestive symptoms – Improves skin problems (acne)[104, 105, 106]

Drink multiple cups a day to enjoy these benefits supported by research. Start by making green or rooibos tea part of your regular beverages of choice.

Want a fun, bubbly drink?

Try mineral water, sparkling water, or even flavored sparkling water (unsweetened). Add fresh berries, or a slice of citrus, other fruit, or cucumber and sweeten with a couple drops of flavored stevia for a sweet refresher. If you're a soda drinker, stevia-sweetened sodas and lightly-sweetened flavored sparkling waters (Zevia®) add some nice variety. They come in an assortment of flavors and are becoming available at most grocery, health, and superstores. Try a couple and find your favorite.

I've shared lots of information in this chapter. Take your time. Digest it. Don't get overwhelmed. Now that we know what to eat for a foundation, let's look more closely at *how* to do it in *your* world.

Be Revitalized

What are the first three changes you will make to your eating?

1.

2.

3.

When will you get started?

What three will come next?

1.

2.

3.

6

How to Make Healthy Doable

Making It Happen

Yes, it is possible to keep it simple and still be delicious. Your new lifestyle need not be complex or cost an arm, leg, and a whole paycheck. If it's too hard, let's face it; we won't do it regularly.

Here are some starting tips to get you mentally prepared and your kitchen prepped so you're set up for success.

1. **Set your goals.**
   - Decide if you'll be going **cold turkey,** all-or-nothing, **OR** if you'll be more slowly and **progressively transitioning** to a new eating lifestyle.

     There's no need to let the changes overwhelm you. Choose what will be **doable and achievable** for you. I personally couldn't handle making all the changes at once. I did what I could. Some was all-or-nothing. Some was a transition. Note: If you're dealing with a serious condition and are miserable with symptoms, the all-or-nothing style will get you on the road to feeling better more quickly. It may be an initial shock, but it's worth it.

- **Be specific and reasonable.** Add more plant-rich, whole foods first. Focusing on what your body needs will naturally fill you up and more easily eliminate empty-calorie foods, pushing out the processed foods, sugars, and large portions of meat and dairy products. Again, you want **attainable goals** that will encourage you along towards health and healing.
- **Write it down.** Whether you use the included *Lifestyle Log* or find an app you prefer, there's something valuable about the accountability of having to record what goes into your mouth. If you're experiencing food sensitivities, this makes it easier to track the potential culprits. Also, taking notes helps greatly with self-awareness. Be sure to track hunger cues and emotions to catch triggers for emotional eating using the *Mindful Eating Journal*. (See Chapter 7 for details.) You can also download a PDF version of all the tracking tools, including the *Grocery Planner,* at InnocentIndulgence.com/TRLtools.
- **Expect results.** You should start to see and experience changes pretty quickly. Everyone is different, but usually within twenty-four to forty-eight hours of making these recommended changes, I get emails from my clients saying, "I can't believe how much better I feel already." Usually renewed energy levels, alertness, pain reduction, and digestive improvements come first.
- **Follow a plan.** Use this guide, or pick just a step or two to get started:

    1. Start by adding in vegetable and fruit servings, which will naturally push out the more prepared (and "fluffy") foods, working up to seven to nine-plus servings daily.
    2. Next, add in adequate water intake.
    3. Monitor and reduce serving sizes.
    4. Switch out your sweeteners from refined and artificial to natural.
    5. Try going gluten-free, if applicable.
    6. Add in omega-3 oils, flaxseeds, and/or chia seeds and focus on good oils.
    7. Switch to grass-fed and free-range meats, eggs, dairy, and nondairy alternatives.

2. **Prepare your kitchen.** This can be as simple or as involved as you'd like it to be. Again, it depends on what results you're looking for, how quickly you want to transition your eating lifestyle, what your body's needs are, and to some extent, the financial investment you are able to make.
    - **Clean out the refrigerator and pantry.** Get rid of anything that will keep you from making the healthiest food choices. Restock with fresh fruits, vegetables, nuts, seeds, grains, herbs and spices, and natural sweeteners, choosing organic foods whenever possible.
    - **Get the right equipment.** A few basic utensils and appliances will help open up a new world of eating. They'll encourage you by helping you save time and energy, and by giving you a better end product. You need the right tools for the job!

- Knife set and sharpener: This is an excellent investment, and don't be afraid of the big knives. They are actually safer and faster, and will produce nicer results once you get comfortable using them.
- Vitamix®, Ninja®, or another high-powered blender with both large and individual containers
- Food processor with various shredding and chopping blades
- Crock-Pot®
- Pots, pans, and bakeware
- Salad spinner—makes washing greens much easier
- Garlic press
- Zester
- Glass, plastic storage containers with lids, and jars of various sizes
- Mixing bowls
- Strainers/sieves
- Meat thermometer
- Spiralizer
- Steamer or a steamer basket
- Electric teapot/kettle
- Juicer (optional) – A press style gives the best-quality juice, but this type is usually more expensive and time-consuming to clean. Centrifugal juicers produce slightly lower-quality juice, but are much easier to clean. Keep in mind that the best-quality juice is the one you actually *make and drink*. (Even an 85 percent quality juice is 100 percent better than none.)

3. **Find new recipes.** A plant-rich, whole-foods lifestyle consists of more than plain salads, veggie sticks, and fruit bowls. In addition to the recipes in this book, other cookbooks and websites will give you delicious recipes to replace traditional dishes. You may even be inspired to

create your own new favorites! Check out the following resources:

- Pinterest, Instagram, and other social media outlets (Be sure to check out InnocentIndulgence.com to get connected)
- AICR.org/healthyrecipes, PCRM.org/health/diets/recipes, or other sites on vegetarian, plant-based eating
- Raw food sites can give excellent, creative ideas for how to prepare veggies

4. **Invest in new dinnerware.** Using **smaller plates, bowls, and glasses will naturally help you keep portion sizes smaller** and retrain your brain as to what a "normal" serving size is (in comparison to our "bottomless" pasta bowls and bread baskets in America). When smaller plates or bowls are full, it feels like you're getting more than when the same amount is served on an oversized plate. On the flip side, be sure you have some fun large plates or bowls for large, main-course salads to help visually retrain your mind regarding your daily produce needs.
5. **Change your meal routine.** Keep serving bowls and food on a buffet line rather than on the table. You can dish up food and snacks, putting away the leftovers *before* eating. These practices will slow down plate refills and overeating.
6. **Open your mind.** Be willing to relearn what popular culture has taught you concerning how to eat. Scientific research supports the wisdom of a whole-foods, plant-rich lifestyle for healing and disease prevention, but grocery stores, food manufacturers, marketing companies, and even some

federal programs want to sell their designer convenience foods. Beware of these traps.

7. **Endure the symptoms of detox.** You may feel a bit worse before you feel better as your body cleans out toxins from years of eating unhealthy, processed food. It will get better, so don't give up. In most cases, give it at least a week. Gluten, as mentioned previously, may take up to six weeks to be flushed from your body, and it can cause withdrawal symptoms. Know it's not just in your head, but that the fatigue, muscle aches, pain, foggy thinking, and low energy will resolve within a few days.
8. **Change your relationship with food.** This topic is a difficult one, and is worthy of a much more in-depth discussion. For now, remember that food is intended for nourishment, fun, and to provide the building blocks for health and protection. But we've been programmed to use food for many other purposes: to celebrate, reward, medicate, comfort, and escape. None of these are totally wrong, but food is meant to be enjoyed in proper balance. Be aware of your relationship with food. Determine where it is unhealthy, and find new, balanced, and creative ways to meet those needs.
9. **Find someone to support you through the process.** You can't do it alone. Whether it's a coach, friend, family member, or spouse, find someone to keep you accountable, to motivate you when you need a kick in the bum, to support you when you feel alone in your choices, to encourage you when you fall off the wagon, and even to do this new life with you. Perhaps the people who don't support

you or who tempt you toward unhealthy habits need to be released, so you can move forward with your goals.

10. **Prepare for this to be a *journey*.** See this as a chance to get rid of the old and to obtain a deeper level of wellness. The destination isn't as important as the journey. Life is all about the process. That's where we change, stretch, grow, and renew. Living a healthy lifestyle is becoming more popular and culturally acceptable. But while many want the results, few are willing to pay the price and make the investment to achieve the health they seek. You can do this! Keep the end goal in mind. Know you're not just doing it for you, but for your family and the many others that you are meant to impact. Many are waiting for you and needing what only *you* have to offer.

Fitting It into Your Wallet and Calendar

Many of my clients find that cost and time constraints are often the biggest concerns in making this transition. So, let's move on to how to minimize your efforts and stretch your dollars:

1. **Simplify.** Meals need not be complicated. Most of us eat the same five to ten meals on a regular basis, over and over. We are creatures of habit, so experiment and decide on a handful of new favorite recipes. Then continue to search for other ideas to add variety and build your recipe base.
2. **Develop a new grocery strategy.** Decide on your new basics and use a list until those ingredients become the norm. Stock up on the new staples for salads, smoothies, dressings, nuts, and whole-grain carbs. Check out the

Grocery Planner provided later in this chapter to use as a starting point.

3. **Choose a few healthy desserts.** This way, when you need a sweet treat, you can make a good decision. This could be anything from fruit "ice cream" (made in the blender) or smoothies to high-percentage (low-sugar) dark chocolate or cookies made with natural sweeteners. Coconut or almond milk ice cream, sweetened with erythritol or cane juice, with peanut butter and chocolate is one of my favorite, convenient standbys. Natural sweeteners give you lots of options for baking (or no bakes) when you have the time.
4. **Buy prewashed greens** and make "instant" salads, smoothies, or juices. (Club stores have great prices on prewashed greens.) Or, prewash your own so they're ready to use when you need them. Sanitize your sink and dunk them all in, using a salad spinner to dry. Store *dry* greens in airtight containers or freshness-extending green bags.
5. **Make smoothies before bed the night before** (especially green smoothies) to speed up morning routines. Store your smoothie in containers of your desired portion, filling jars completely and leaving no air space. This limits oxidation and maximizes nutrition. Alternatively, preload an individual-sized blender cup to help you make a quick morning getaway with a fresh blend on the go. Greens can even be frozen and premade into "smoothie kits." Just pop prepped ingredients into the blender and add last-minute liquids or ice just before blending.

6. **Make a couple of your favorite soups (and beans) in large batches**, and freeze some for another time. Plan to make enough for at least two extra meals.
7. **Use your Crock-Pot®.** This is such a great way to prepare large quantities of soup, stew, beans, or meat with little monitoring. Dinner can be ready for you when you walk in the door!
8. **Stock up.** Make storage space available so you have what you need, either in cold storage or the pantry.
9. **Buy in bulk and freeze** to save money. Shop at co-ops, club stores, and online. Club stores offer great deals on large quantities of produce (fresh and frozen) and organic meat. Package fresh fruit, raw or even cooked meats and freeze, dividing into meal-sized or useable recipe portions until you're ready to use. (Use caution, as some foods should not be refrozen once thawed.)
10. **Prepare meat in bulk** by grilling, baking, frying, or slow cooking, and freeze it so you can quickly add it to salads, soups, wraps, or other veggie-based entrées.
11. **Portion large-batch recipes to be frozen into meal-sized servings** for faster thawing and reheating, and to prevent waste. This works great for soups, stews, beans, leftover baked dishes, cooked meats and more.
12. **Plan for leftovers to give you double meals.** This will help stretch your time. If you reheat slowly and add a little water if needed, you'll never know the meals aren't freshly made. Serve dressings or sauces on the side to keep salads and veggies crisp, and to keep meats from getting soggy.

13. **Use some convenience foods.** Canned beans are great. Be sure to rinse and drain them well to make them more easily digestible and to reduce the sodium content. Packaged ground flaxseed meal may not have 100 percent of the nutrition that freshly ground does, but even a 10 percent loss in freshness gives you 90 percent more than nothing.
14. **Load up your office and commuting bag with preportioned snacks and bottled water.** Having good snacks available keeps your energy up and reduces the temptation of empty-calorie snacking. Keeping water with you makes it easier to stay hydrated and to prevent confusion of hunger and thirst cues from your body.
15. **Find a fun or pretty glass** to make drinking water throughout the day more exciting. Fill your bottle or jug with water several times a day and make goals to finish it by lunch, midafternoon, or bedtime so you can get in your daily hydration needs.
16. **Grow your own herbs.** The fresh, bright flavor of herbs can really make salads, veggies, soups, and meat come to life. Fresh cilantro, basil, chives, garlic, peppers, mint, and even stevia are amazing! Plus, growing herbs is an easy intro to gardening.
17. **Plant a garden.** You can't beat the freshness and flavor of homegrown produce! Many plants will grow in a window box, in a pot on the porch, in a corner of the yard, or even in a small, raised garden. You'll get hooked! Somehow, it's more exciting to be involved in what you eat when you grow it yourself. And having a garden can even get kids more

excited about veggies. Gardening is also a relaxing and refreshing way to enjoy sunshine and fresh air. For a successful garden, be sure to explore recommended planting times, sunlight needs, soil blends, most successful seeds and/or varieties, fertilizer, water schedules, and organic pest control for your area.

18. **Visit farmers' markets or U-Pick farms.** Although these can be more expensive, in-season fruits and veggies grown locally give you higher nutrient content and flavor. They also make great outings for families and friends.
19. **Try new stores and brands.** You may need to grocery-store-hop to find more variety, your new favorite items, and the best prices. Big-name stores are not always less expensive. Sometimes mom-and-pop health shops have unique specialty items at even lower prices. Check online too, as there are unlimited options, and often, you can get better prices for larger quantities and free shipping.
20. **Skip the beverage.** Choose water when eating out, or choose only a beverage, sides, and an appetizer.
21. **Split meals.** Most restaurant portions are enough for more than one person. Splitting a meal helps to cut costs, portions, and that miserable overstuffed feeling.
22. **Eat out during lunch or happy hour.** Lunch or happy hour menu selections usually offer lighter portions and better prices.

Meal and Snack Starters

Here are some ideas to help you redesign your menus for nutrient density and delicious flavors.

Meals

- Wraps using whole grain, corn, sprouted tortillas, or lettuce wraps (use stiffer or flexible greens: butter lettuce, chard, collards, kale, romaine, cabbage) stuffed with chopped veggies, a spread, and your choice of protein (nitrite/nitrate-, hormone-, and chemical-free deli sliced chicken, turkey, grass-fed beef, or wild fish).
  - Butter lettuce, tomatoes, sprouts, avocado, mushrooms, spicy mustard
  - Romaine, tomatoes, cucumber, onions, green peppers, hummus
  - Tortilla, spinach, zucchini, olives, onions, garlic, sun-dried tomatoes, Italian seasoning, fresh herbs
  - Romaine, tomatoes, garlic, peppers, onions, guacamole, beans
- Large salad combo ideas:
  - **Mexican**: Romaine, tomatoes, avocado, onions, garlic, peppers, black or kidney beans, cilantro with lime juice and/or salsa with corn tortillas or baked tortilla chips
  - **Greek**: Spinach, tomatoes, cucumber, Kalamata olives, onions, feta, garlic, Italian seasoning, oregano, basil, lemon juice or balsamic vinegar, and olive oil

- **Seasonal sweet**: Adding fruit (apples, oranges, raisins, berries, pomegranate) and nuts balance flavors of darker greens and give the salad a great crunch
- **Grilled Veggie Fajita Salad**: Lightly steamed or stir-fried veggies (peppers, onions, broccoli, squash, zucchini, carrots, mushrooms) on greens
- **Kale**: Lemon, olive oil, and garlic work great for a dressing, or skip the garlic and add fruit or a splash of fruit juice
- **Asian**: Cabbage or greens base, carrots, peppers, onions, mushrooms, nuts (almonds, cashews, peanuts), pineapple or mango with sesame/tamari dressing or lime juice, basil, cilantro
- **Cabbage or slaws**: Green cabbage, onions and carrots with mayo-based dressing OR purple cabbage, onions, cilantro with slightly sweetened, creamy lime juice dressing
- **Other tips**:
  - Choose dressings with "good fats" (e.g., olive oil, flaxseed oil)
  - Avoid partially hydrogenated oils and sugars
  - Add beans (black, kidney, garbanzo)
  - Add sunflower or pumpkin seeds or other nuts

• Baked spaghetti squash or stir-fried zucchini (instead of traditional pasta) topped with marinara sauce, sun-dried tomatoes, or fire-roasted tomatoes
  - Add mushrooms, onions, or even broccoli for a veggie boost

- Black beans and rice with chopped onion, tomato, and avocado
  - Add salsa, cilantro, and peppers, or simplify by topping with guacamole
- Soups or stews loaded with veggies and beans
- Steamed broccoli or cauliflower topped with minced onions, garlic, olive oil, reduced-sodium tamari, and even nutritional yeast
  - Serve larger portions in a big bowl
  - If cheese makes it go down more easily, add an organic variety
- Steamed veggies (e.g., green beans, carrots) tossed with olive oil or organic butter, sea salt, and seasonings
  - Sprinkle zucchini with a touch of garlic
  - Add ginger to carrots
- Green beans stir-fried with slivered almonds and steak seasoning, or simmered with onions, diced red potato, mushrooms, and clean, smoked turkey
- Layered baked dishes or casseroles with added veggies
  - Baked squash and/or zucchini with black beans, peppers, onions, and cheddar, topped with crumbled, baked multigrain or corn chips served with salsa and avocado or guacamole
  - Zucchini or veggie lasagna
  - Chicken and veggie enchilada bake
- Baked sweet potatoes (yams) topped with cinnamon, apples or unsweetened applesauce, raisins, and walnuts or pecans

- Baked butternut squash seasoned with olive oil or butter and seasonings of choice (e.g., sea salt, cinnamon, garlic, nutmeg)
- Stuff peppers, mushrooms, or tomatoes with veggies, guacamole, beans, brown rice, and protein (tuna, turkey, chicken, or grass-fed beef)
- Stir-fried veggie blends: broccoli, cauliflower, peppers, carrots, snow peas, mushrooms, and chard or spinach, garlic, and ginger with coconut aminos (or tamari), teriyaki or other Asian sauces
- Green smoothies work great as either a meal or snack

Add your choice of protein to any of these for variety.

Snacks

- Apple or banana slices with 100 percent natural nut butter (e.g., cashew, almond, peanut), sprinkled with cinnamon and raisins
- Whole grain or sprouted tortillas
  - Top with nut butter and honey or 100 percent fruit spread
  - Make wraps filled with veggies, sauce, dip, or spread
- Hummus, bean, or vegetable dip with veggies (mini peppers, grape tomatoes, carrots, celery, cucumbers, broccoli, cauliflower, sugar snap peas, and more)
- Salsa, guacamole, and/or bean dip with baked corn chips or veggies (jicama, cucumbers, squash, cauliflower)
- Fresh fruit or fruit salads
- Celery with nut butter, livened up with cinnamon and raisins
- Raw nuts or trail mix

- Frozen fruit topped with a vanilla milk alternative (almond, coconut) and natural sweetener
- Walnuts, raisins, and apple slices
- Smoothies or fruit shakes
- Peanut butter-chocolate-banana shake
- Naked popcorn or seasoned with nutritional yeast and sea salt
- Kale chips
- Flax chips
- Crispy, roasted chickpeas

Shopping Guide

Finding and identifying these new treasures and expanding into new foods can be overwhelming, especially when it comes to shopping. Use the following label-reading tips and *Grocery Planner* for ideas and directions on picking tasty choices and starting your own new grocery list. (Note: the *Grocery Planner* is not an exhaustive list, but one to help expand your ideas and creativity. Download a PDF version at InnocentIndulgence.com/TRLtools.)

Label Reading

Here are a few tips to simplify decoding food labels in order to find out what's *really* in your food:

- **Find the sugar content.** Remember, sugar has many other names in ingredient lists. Look for items with natural sweeteners when possible, especially avoiding high fructose corn syrup. Then, calculate sugar content. In the Total

Carbohydrate section, you'll notice that it lists Sugars. Four grams of sugar equals one teaspoon. For example, sixteen grams of sugar equals four teaspoons of sugar or 4 sugar packets. If you have a high total carb count, be sure the item has fiber to slow the rise of blood sugars.

- **Check the fiber content.** For carb-heavy foods, look for items with *at least* three grams of fiber (the amount can be located under Total Carbohydrates). The higher the number, the better. Incorporate high-fiber foods like beans, vegetables, fruit, grains, flax and chia seeds into your diet in order to get your daily thirty to forty grams of fiber.
- **Examine for trans fats.** Labeling laws allow for foods with less than half a gram of trans fats to be labeled as "trans-fat-free," so be sure to look for hydrogenated fats in the ingredient list. If it's on the label, trans fats *are* present. As a side note, omega-3s are not required to be labeled, so often you'll only see them listed on a label if an item is specifically being marketed for omega-3 benefits.
- **Go low sodium.** Packaged foods usually have way too much sodium. Choose items that use sea salt and have the lowest possible sodium count. Limit items that contain 400+ milligrams per serving.
- **Note serving sizes.** Beverages are especially famous for splitting a large can or bottle into two or three servings. If this is the case, adjust your serving size to fit the label, or multiply the numbers to fit the amount you actually consume.
- **Pronounce the ingredient list.** If you are struggling to say the words, the product is likely to be highly processed

with lots of additives and/or preservatives. Look for another option. Shorter lists and simple ingredients are usually better, cleaner choices.

- **Consider the calories.** Although I'm not a calorie counter and I rarely talk about calories, it is important to be aware of how many calories are going into your body. Check out the calorie counts for fancy coffee drinks and restaurant entrées to get a few big surprises.

Grocery Planner

Veggies

Asparagus
Broccoli
Brussels sprouts
Cauliflower
Celery
Tomatoes
Green beans
Peas (baby, snap)
Cabbage (green, red)
Bok choy
Napa cabbage
Chard (green, rainbow)
Kale (dino, curly)
Spinach
Butter lettuce
Romaine
Green/red leaf lettuce
Mushrooms
Onions
Leeks
Scallions
Garlic (fresh, powder, dried)
Peppers (red, yellow, green, orange, hot)
Beets
Carrots
Parsnips
Potatoes (red, gold)
Radishes
Turnips
Sweet potatoes
Yams
Cucumber
Eggplant
Summer squash
Zucchini
Winter squash
Spaghetti squash
Butternut squash
Acorn squash

Fruit

Apples
Pears
Pomegranates
Bananas
Blackberries
Blueberries
Raspberries
Strawberries
Loganberries
Cranberries
Cantaloupe
Honeydew
Watermelon
Pumpkin
Figs
Dates
Dried fruit
Grapes
Lemons
Limes
Oranges
Grapefruit
Tangerines
Rhubarb
Apricots
Cherries
Nectarines
Peaches
Plums
Pineapple
Papayas
Mangos
Kiwis

Beans

Black beans
Black-eyed peas
Cannellini beans
Garbanzo beans
Great northern beans
Lentils
Kidney beans

Pinto beans
Split peas
Navy beans

Oils
Avocado oil
Coconut oil
Olive oil
Flaxseed oil
Flaxseed
Chia seed
Sesame oil

Nuts/Seeds
Almonds
Brazil
Cashews
Hazelnuts
Pecans
Pine nuts
Macadamia nuts
Pistachios
Peanuts
Walnuts
Nut butters (almond, cashew, peanut, tahini)
Pumpkin seeds
Sunflower seeds

Grains
Amaranth
Buckwheat
Millet
Quinoa
Rice (wild, brown, basmati)
Cornmeal (organic)
Oats
Einkorn wheat
Coconut flour
Nut flour/meal

Natural Sweeteners
Stevia (powder, liquid, flavored)
Raw honey
Maple syrup
Coconut sugar
Xylitol

Protein
Beef (lean, grass-fed) Chicken, turkey (cage-free)
Wild fish
Eggs (omega-3, free-range)
Cheeses (organic)
Yogurt (organic, unsweetened)
—all hormone free

Beverages
Tea (green, herbal, black, rooibos)
Sparkling water
Zevia®

Milk Alternatives
Almond, Coconut, Coconut creamer

Flavorings
Basil
Cilantro
Cinnamon
Cloves
Curry
Cumin
Ginger
Italian seasoning
Mint
Mustard
Oregano
Parsley
Pepper (black, red flakes)
Rosemary
Sea salt
Vinegar (coconut, apple cider, balsamic)
Coconut aminos
Tamari—low sodium Cocoa
Coconut
Extracts (lemon, vanilla, almond)

Dining Out and Parties

Whether it's for a stay-cation, vacation, business trip, or just eating on the go, dining out is often the most convenient—and the most tempting—when it comes to veering off track from healthy lifestyle eating. But with a few, easy tweaks to your menu perusing, you can creatively make choices to keep you feeling—and eating—your best.

1. **Spruce up your drinks.** Water and tea provide better hydration, especially during the summer months, and can be transformed with lemon, lime, orange, berries, or cucumber slices. Sweeten coffee and teas with stevia or a bit of raw honey. Cinnamon also adds a sweet flavor and makes coffee a special treat without the sugar. While traveling, stuff a few stevia packets or a travel-sized flavored stevia bottle in your bag and share them with friends. If you want to splurge for sweetened coffee drinks, request half or even one-quarter of the normal amount of syrup pumps. You'll be surprised how yummy it still is!
2. **Think twice on the appetizers.** Skip deep-fried treats and rich, creamy dips, which are full of extra (bad) fats with little nutrition. Lettuce wraps or other veggie plates make great starters. Or, request a fresh veggie plate alongside hummus or other dips instead of chips, pitas, and other "fluffy" calories.
3. **Build your own entrée.** Survey the menu for available items, and request your own custom-designed salads, stir-frys, entrées, and sides. Wait staff love it when you call it the "Waiter/Waitress's name Special." Besides, most chefs

love the extra challenge, and it often comes out a little fresher and better.

4. **Add veggies.** Whether it's a pizza, sandwich, or pasta dish, add some fresh veggies to get a nutrient and flavor boost. Steamed veggies make a great replacement for pasta, veggie pizzas are terrific (and beautiful), and wraps can help reduce the "fluff."
5. **Keep it "lite."** Request your dressings and sauces on the side to reduce unnecessary fat intake. A little dab will go a long way to enhance flavor. Order "no oil" or "light oil" for stir-frys, omelets, eggs, fajitas, and other fried foods, which can be cooked deliciously without being oil-soaked.
6. **Skip the refills.** Keep the bread and chip baskets to one per visit (unless you're part of a large party). It's easy to mindlessly fill up on chips and bread before your meal even comes, especially if you're hungry.
7. **Make it 100 percent fruit.** If you're choosing a smoothie, request only real fruit, not juice or a fruit-juice concentrate that's been processed (lower fiber and nutrients with higher sugar). Request a milk alternative, coconut water, water, or ice as a substitute for fruit juice.
8. **Split a meal.** Whether you take half your meal home for a second meal or share with a friend, using this tactic will reduce your portion size. America is known for supersizing!
9. **Monitor your trips.** Buffets and family-style dining can make it easy to overeat. Set your limits beforehand. Start with green salads or other veggie dishes, and finish off with sampler-sized portions of entrées.

10. **Ask and inform.** Whether you call ahead or discuss it when you sit down at the table, make sure your waiter knows of any special food restrictions, allergies, or sensitivities to head off potential reactions, cross-contaminations, or frustrating do-overs. Be sure they understand and are able to accommodate your requests.
11. **Research.** If you have specific preferences, a few minutes of research or a couple of calls can make you and your party much happier. Restaurants that serve special meals, gluten-free, vegetarian/vegan, and plant-based options are exploding in popularity.

Enjoy your dining experience! Kick back, unwind, laugh, and make memories with those special people. And keep the food as an accent, not the main feature to your time of relaxation.

Travel and On-the-Run Eating

With our highly-mobilized society, away-from-home food choices are important. Whether you're on a road trip, an outdoor adventure with family or friends, off for business travels, making a long commute, or just needing to grab something between meetings, here are a few ways to make better food choices that your body will love.

1. **Pack up simple snacks or no-prep food.** While on a road trip, minimize the fast food/convenience mart/truck stop (and totally empty-calorie!) munchies with some of these:

Fresh fruit	Kale chips
Hummus and veggies	Lightly sweetened granola
Fresh and dried fruit	Whole-food bars
Raw nuts	Roasted chickpeas
Trail mix	Nut butters
Popcorn	

2. **Nibble on preportioned snacks.** Choose small packages and make your own snack bags, or just close the bag to help prevent mindless eating during long hours on the road.
3. **Bring picnic snacks or meals.** Invest in an insulated lunch bag or cooler (and ice packs) to keep foods cold and prevent foodborne illness. This also lowers the travel budget.
4. **Research before you go.** Look into the area's food culture, and find local restaurants that have healthier options. Most hotels also have in-room refrigerators available, allowing for a local farmers' market or grocery store run. Stock up on snack items or easy meals (especially breakfast). For specific food selections, restrictions or sensitivities, call ahead to make special arrangements with theme parks, airlines, conference meals, or even hotel dining.
5. **Study menus.** Build a "custom" entrée using menu ingredients listed. Chefs usually love the challenge, quite often building you something that everyone else will wish they had ordered!
6. **Stick to your normal food schedule.** Keep meals light to even out your energy levels and to avoid the "I'm starving" binges on foods or portions you would not normally choose.

7. **Hydrate.** Drink plenty of water to keep you feeling good, having fun, and thinking clearly. Buy it by the gallon or the travel bottle. Remember, altitude and low humidity on planes easily dehydrate you and make jet lag worse. Drink at least eight ounces of water per hour, and avoid caffeine and alcohol. Be sure to drink *at least* an extra two to three cups of water on travel days.
8. **Splurge . . . in moderation.** It's vacation! Of course you're going to want to eat more "special" food. Just remember to split it or go with the smaller size. Most importantly, pay attention to how you feel afterwards (e.g., tired, low energy, cranky, agitated, energized, stuffed, miserable), asking yourself, "Was it really worth it?" The time will come when it becomes "worth it" less and less often.
9. **Sip wisely.** Choose unsweetened or lightly sweetened beverages. Try various herbal teas with honey, or club soda with lime. Sweet coffee drinks, soft drinks, or other "adult beverages" are usually full of empty calories that add up quickly, especially during vacations. Smaller sizes help avoid excess "liquid calories," many of which also dehydrate the body.
10. **Exercise.** Whether you're spending a long day in meetings or in a car, plane, or train, you'll feel much better if you get your blood circulating. Take a five-to-ten-minute walk at rest stops. Walk the length of the plane every hour or so. Explore the area around your hotel for fifteen to twenty minutes. Or squeeze in a short swim or a trip to your accommodation's gym if you prefer.

Have a great time, and make happy memories of the excursions, sights, and sounds with your coworkers, family, or friends. Love the food, but keep it as a highlight, not the primary focus of the trip.

Holiday Trimmings

It's the most wonderful time of the year! The Christmas holiday is one of my favorite seasons with the lights, nostalgia, time with family and friends, crisp air, dreams of "White Christmases," cozy fires, candles, rich colors, the precious significance, and of course, fabulous flavors. Mid-November through the first week of January can be one big holiday party. Within our extended family, we have four birthdays during this time, in addition to Thanksgiving, at least two Christmases, and have even taken part in Hanukkah celebrations. And, that doesn't even count the other seasonal parties, get-togethers, and shopping sprees that include my favorite seasonal flavors, coffees, and goodies.

So, what do holidays look like when you're living a lifestyle of health? How can you survive the season without requiring a crash recovery course on January 2? Here are the secrets I've learned that can help you make holidays, birthday, parties, and special occasions enjoyable and healthful.

1. **Start now.** It doesn't matter. Even if you're in the middle of the holiday season. Start today and begin reaping the benefits of making even little lifestyle changes. It's not too late, and sometimes beginning "tomorrow" doesn't seem to happen.

2. **Be realistic.** There's no need to plan for weight loss from November to December; just plan to maintain, not gain.
3. **Eat breakfast.** Skipping meals typically sets you up to fail later in the day, making you hungrier and more likely to fill up on the abundant holiday treats. Plus, breakfast is the perfect time to fit in green smoothies to help balance out whatever choices come later in the day.
4. **Stay active.** Your gym routine, walk, or jog may be shortened, but some exercise is still better than none. The holidays are the perfect time of year to enjoy a brisk walk, to look at lights, to try ice-skating, or to do a short, home workout.
5. **Plan ahead.** If you know you're going to a party, balance the rest of your day's eating accordingly. Eat lighter, plant-rich, nutrient-dense foods before the event. Limit yourself to a single trip through the food line. Have a snack (a green smoothie, veggie plate, or salad) before you go in order to reduce the party munchies.
6. **Sip wisely.** Lattes, hot chocolate, cider, and other party drinks are usually loaded with empty calories and have little nutritional value. These drinks can easily lead to weight gain, especially when paired with other holiday goodies. Choose stevia or honey to sweeten hot beverages, sip sparkling waters, or use stevia-sweetened sodas as a base for your mixed beverages. You can also try stevia-sweetened bubbling ciders. Pick your favorite indulgent drinks in moderation.
7. **Try new recipes.** Look for simple recipes from the endless possibilities on social media. Just a few simple

modifications can tweak your favorites into healthful deliciousness, while experimenting with a few new ingredients can hook you on new favorites.

8. **Make and freeze ahead.** Make a big pot of veggie- or bean-based soup or stew to freeze for a quick, nourishing meal during time crunches later in the month.
9. **Stay hydrated.** This will keep thirst cues from being confused with hunger cues, and will keep you feeling more full and satisfied. Staying hydrated will also keep you sharp, focused, and energized throughout the holiday season.
10. **Add to the party.** If you can, take a "healthy version" dish or snack to contribute to the party spread. Share the goodness, and know you will have a good option to enjoy.
11. **Hide or freeze the goodies.** While you know where they are, keeping sweets out of sight does slow down the nibbles, compared to seeing them out on the counter, in the cookie jar, or in a candy bowl.
12. **Create your own coffees.** Most peppermint mochas, eggnog lattes and other specialty holiday coffees are loaded with sugar and artificial ingredients. Home coffee systems are becoming popular, which allow you to make your own coffees easily, with clean ingredients, and free of processed sugars. Use flavored coffee beans or spice up the blend on your own. Add a natural sweetener and froth an unsweetened milk alternative for a heavenly (and virtually no-calorie) drink.
13. **Be still.** In the midst of the bustle, take a few minutes to slow down and unwind. The holidays can be very busy and stressful. Light candles and turn on decorative lights,

listen to Christmas music, and just "be" to clear your mind, refocus, relax, and ponder the real meaning of the season.

14. **Slow down.** The December calendar can easily be overloaded with programs, concerts, parties, shopping, family events, and a host of other special activities. But you don't have to get caught up in chaotic schedules. Choose the events that are most important. Simplify traditions. Be creative. Decorations can be just as beautiful and meals just as delicious when simply done. Your friends and family will likely appreciate the reduced pressures too.
15. **Enjoy the season.** Go ahead and indulge in a piece of pumpkin pie, a couple of gingerbread cookies, or whatever your favorite goodies may be, choosing reasonable portions. Savor the memories, traditions, and special times with those you hold dear. Be in the moment, love every bite, and don't feel guilty!
16. **Celebrate your victories.** Focus on the progress you make in the season. Whether it's maintaining an exercise routine, trying new recipes, reducing sweet beverages, or avoiding the extra holiday pounds, congratulate yourself! Remember, every single step forward counts.

Wherever you may be and whatever season of life you're in, choose to make this holiday season your best one yet. Marvel at the beauty, ponder the significance, and savor the Goodness of the Season.

Now, let's look at how you can stay motivated in the dailies on this new journey.

Be Revitalized

What three tips will you put into action to make this daily journey easier for you and your unique lifestyle?

1.

2.

3.

7

How to Stay Motivated

Let's face it. You're likely to fall off the wagon a time or two . . . or twenty . . . or 120! It's OK. Get up and start again. It's not all or nothing. Every single step forward is making a difference.

According to research in neuroscience, **it takes a total of sixty-three days to fully and completely change a habit, so be sure to allow yourself grace and breaks**. The first twenty-one days help you to move a short-term memory into long-term memory, but it requires two more twenty-one day cycles (forty-two more days) to make it "automatic."[107] This is a *big* change—huge, in fact! You're likely reprogramming an entire lifetime of eating, so it isn't going to happen overnight, or maybe not even after sixty-three days. Reprogramming your eating habits will require discipline and focus. It also takes time for your taste buds to adapt and to begin correlating how you eat relates to how you feel. What's more, many of these eating and lifestyle changes are still somewhat countercultural, so your decision will have to be stable and unchanging even when it means going against the "norm." It may seem a high price to pay, but the results are priceless.

Before you start your journey, fill out the *Symptom Tracker* at the end of the book. Note every symptom, ache, pain, discomfort, and energy-level variation you are experiencing, and rate them on a scale of zero (nothing) to five (awful or frequent).

After three or four weeks of your new eating lifestyle, go back through that list and re-rate those same points. Surprised at the difference? Look for changes in energy, pain levels, or symptoms. Notice the difference in how foods taste. Some things probably taste brighter and more vibrant. Fruit may seem sweeter, greens and vegetables may be less bitter, sweets might taste too sweet, while some foods may now be too salty. You might begin to pick up the taste of pesticides, food additives or even the now noticeable blandness of nonorganic produce. Then, compare how you're feeling *after* eating well to how you felt *after* the time(s) of "falling off the wagon." Quite a difference, right? Your energy levels can drop, pain levels can increase, digestive symptoms can flare, and thinking can get foggy. But soon, there will come a time when going back to the old ways won't be worth it to you. You'll naturally prefer feeling good and making choices that keep you feeling that way.

Remember that this is not a rigid, end-all plan. It's **a guideline for the "dailies."** Let's face it. Life happens. Best intentions don't transpire. Unexpected circumstances pop up. Opportunities to travel for business or pleasure arise. Holidays, moving, babies, advanced schooling, and other unique seasons of life happen. **Each time of life has its own unique needs and will require something a little different for you to be at your best**.

The key is being aware of what your body needs in each season and doing your best to make it happen. You may need a detox season. You may need a rebuilding season. You may need a "relaxed" season. And thankfully, grocery stores and restaurants are becoming more accommodating to health-conscious shoppers and diners, which makes this process easier and more convenient. Stick to what's best for your body while still enjoying your current season.

It's Not All About the Food

If only eating specific foods in specific amounts in a specific way were enough to make everything fall easily into place. But while nutrition and a healthy lifestyle are essential pieces to health, **true wellness is much deeper and nutrition is only one part of the solution.** The CDC reports, "Eighty-three percent of all deaths for adults between the ages of 21 and 65 are related to lifestyle," which include "our environmental and societal pressures," and "our competitive, success-oriented way of life."[108,109,110] In fact, 75 to 90 percent of doctors' visits are related to *stress*.[111]

We've been so intricately put together in a way that does not allow us to compartmentalize our physical, emotional, and spiritual elements. Each piece affects the other. Stress is a perfect example of the body, mind, and spirit connection. When we're stressed, our worried thoughts and belief systems affect our physical bodies. Loss of appetite, indigestion, muscle tension, headaches, heart palpitations, shaking, and sleeplessness are just a few, as **stress (specifically fear) causes over 1,400 physical and chemical changes in the body**.[112] Even more intriguing is the fact that our bodies can't tell the difference between being chased by a lion, facing a pressing deadline, or dealing with a relationship conflict. Each of these different events registers as stress, and our "fight or flight" mechanism kicks in, affecting all of the body's systems.

How do we deal with such high levels of stress? For a majority of us, it noticeably affects our eating. While 36 percent of women and 23 percent of men skip meals, the *American Psychological Association* reports 43 percent of women and 32 percent of men say they overeat or eat unhealthy foods due to stress, with about half of them cycling in this behavior at least weekly.[113] **Emotional eating is a huge, complicated dynamic**, often implicated through culture. Generations of family food patterns, marketing from food companies, and even our finances and the economy all play a role in our emotional eating. I see it all the time, and I've experienced it myself. I love it when science puts numbers to our daily lives. According to neuroscientist Dr. Caroline Leaf, **nutrition is only about 20 percent of the healthy-lifestyle picture, while up to 80 percent is dependent on what we're *thinking***. What's going on inside our heads affects everything from our food selections, to digestion, to the absorption of nutrients, and to our overall health.[114]

So, *why* are you really eating? Studies that look at the success of emotional awareness are beginning to emerge. Findings indicate that **those who learn emotional awareness are more likely to be successful and achieve healthier weights, drop excess weight or prevent weight gain**.[115] Even those feeling "hopeful toward the future" tended to make better food choices than those who had negative mindsets.[116]

We're often subconsciously driven by painful situations from our pasts, which can translate into poor health and food choices at stores and restaurants, in the kitchen, at meal times . . . and every time in-between. So again, *why are you really eating*? Because you're hungry? Because it's lunchtime and everyone else is eating?

Or, **are you really eating just because you are actually *feeling something***? Maybe you're experiencing one of the common triggers associated with emotional eating:

Stressed	Sad	Guilty
Tired	Afraid	Frustrated
Happy	Confused	Rejected
Lonely	Overwhelmed	Jealous
Bored	Embarrassed	Ashamed
Angry	Shy	Worried
Anxious	Left out	Hopeful
Ignored	Hysterical	Irritable
Depressed	Exhausted	Numb

Or, *how hungry are you really?* Are you actually *thirsty* instead of hungry? Many times, we don't properly assess hunger and thirst signals because we are so caught up in our emotions and the patterns and habits we use to manage them. We must get in tune with what our bodies and hearts are telling us, so we can make wise choices to meet the real needs. **Food isn't the answer—especially to fill emotional needs**. You may need to ask yourself, **"What's eating me?"** Get to the root and look at what is going on inside. How's your heart? What are you truly (although maybe subconsciously) thinking about or believing? This affects not only the foods you choose to eat, but ultimately your physical health. Check out the *Mindful Eating Journal* at the back of the book to increase your awareness of emotional eating patterns, to become conscious of better ways of processing them, and to address them before they escalate.

A physical need or condition is a short-term motivator as we become desperate to relieve the pain, weight, or other symptoms. When the symptoms get bad enough, we're willing to do almost anything to stop the misery. But many times, this is still not enough. **I've had clients eating perfectly, yet their symptoms remained, quite often because of unresolved emotional pain, trauma, grief, or a repressed loss.**

The same was true for me. I was eating perfectly and was getting some relief, but then I hit a plateau. Many of my symptoms were controlled but not resolved. But things really started to change when I slowed down and took a deeper look into my heart and mind. I began to be honest with myself about my thoughts and feelings, facing the things I had repressed and stuffed away over the years. I didn't like what I saw: buried childhood hurts that my young heart had recorded and carried as trauma for years, the pain of lost love and friends, hidden bitterness and resentment toward abusive educational, business, and personal relationships, unhealthy patterns that had been passed down through the generations in my family, dark layers of fear and disappointment, and ugly places of shame and self-hatred. These all contributed to a lack of vision, passion, and hope for my future.

I even found that my faith was surprisingly shallow. Though I had grown up around a strong faith and one that I'm ever so thankful was deeply grounded in Truth, I realized I hadn't made it my own. It had been merely a religion, a system of "doing things right" that was built on a belief *about* God instead of *knowing and experiencing* who He really is: Healer, Father, Friend, Comforter, Love, Power, and Hope, just to name a few. I had made my faith into a list of religious things to *do* or *not do*, and that by these works, I could please Him and earn His love, instead of belief, trust and intimacy with a God who loved *me*. Instead, I thought of Him as a distant, unloving, weak God who was the main character of a book of stories that somehow didn't seem to have relevancy for today. I was settling for way less than what was available to me, with a form of powerless religion that left me empty and with a broken, distorted image of God.

A series of events and circumstances brought me to a turning point. A friend (and very successful business owner) with a similar faith background shared how he had just returned from co-leading a healing trip to India, resulting in miraculous stories of children unable to see, hear, or talk being completely healed. I was shocked. I could see he was not simply talking about a distant, religious God, but One who he seemed to know in a different way. He was experiencing and demonstrating a God of love, healing, and power that I hadn't even known existed. I *knew* then that those stories weren't just from a book for long ago, but for *today* . . . and for *me*. My friend then prayed for healing for me, and from that day forward, the debilitating fatigue lifted. It was a miraculous turn of events, in more ways than one.

As time passed, I began to face each of my hurts and false belief systems, letting them go. I forgave others and myself, detoxing from unhealthy thought patterns and emotions, and opening my heart and mind to heal. I relearned what was true about life, others, myself, and especially the One who was the true source of the love, hope, destiny, peace, comfort, and friendship that I so needed.

More healing and freedom came as the dark layers were exposed, resolved, and peeled off. Refreshing and peace set in. New hope sprang up. Healthier patterns of thinking and living replaced toxic ones. Passions were uncovered and dreams were birthed, launching me in new directions. I *really* began to see the results I had been waiting for, and the symptoms I'd been experiencing for so long started to disappear. I'm happy to say, I am the healthiest, freest, and most "well" I have ever been in my life since walking down this road. Was it easy? Not exactly. But once you get a taste of the healing, freedom, and life that is available for you, you won't want to settle for anything less.

Everyone's journey is different. Each of us is unique, with different talents, gifts, interests, purposes, callings, families, upbringings, and life experiences. But, we all experience pain, trauma, and grief. We all experience loss in some form, whether it's the loss of health, family, friends, relationships, jobs, finances, innocence, dreams, direction, purpose, or even hope. Each of these can be excruciatingly painful. And oftentimes, they begin happening when we're young and incapable of processing adult circumstances through a child's perceptions. But, **if these things are not dealt with properly, the emotional pain remains and eventually creates harmful physical and emotional effects**. This is why we must let go of the past, forgive, and move forward to enjoy clean living in every area of life—including our belief systems about ourselves, others, and the world around us.

Tasting Real Health…and Hope

Touching on this deep subject is outside the ordinary scope of a nutrition text, but I wanted to share about what has been so *pivotal* to my healing and that of many others I've met. I've seen physical healing occur time after time when the emotional and spiritual blockages to health are removed. I have friends and know of others healed of multiple sclerosis, schizophrenia, fibromyalgia, life-threatening lung conditions, nearsightedness, horrific abuses and traumas, and so much more. It really is the foundation for wellness, but it is often the piece that isn't discussed or explored. **The true change and motivation that we need in order to achieve health and success in life must begin from within.** Our spirit and soul need to be just as well-nourished as our physical body.

This is why knowing your true value and worth is so essential. It goes to the core of who you are, what you believe about yourself, and therefore, life. Women especially, seem to struggle with low self-worth, looking to culture, a significant other, family, kids, jobs, and food to fill their longing for love and meaning. Men are no different, but they hide it better and have a little less pressure from culture and the media. Go back with me to your childhood dreams of being a princess or a valiant, warrior prince (or superhero), the days when you were beautiful or handsome, carefree, confident, powerful, victorious, and at peace. Who told you that you weren't a princess? And that you couldn't be the princess rescued and swept off into the sunset by the prince? Or, the hero prince who comes to rescue the lovely princess and conquer the kingdom? **The truth is, this is who you *really are meant to be*!** Ladies, you *are* that beautiful princess. You really can be clean, pure, and perfect, and can experience the radiant life you've thought was only a dream. You are meant to have a passionate influence and powerful voice to our culture through the unique beauty and creativity *you* bring to the world—through art and design, business, speaking, caregiving, etc. Men, you really can be the brave warrior that conquers land and the fearless leader that guides and protects the princess, heirs (family), and territory (business, government, and more). Those dreams of significance were put there by your King, the Lover of your heart and your Creator, who wants to make them come true for you in a way you can't possibly imagine.

Daily life, painful circumstances, and the evil enemy of our hearts are what make us think those dreams are just fairytales beyond our reach. What if we were to believe in those dreams and live out the truths of our identity, knowing that we are . . . as a beautiful bride or a bold warrior . . . leaders and influencers—courageous, powerful, victorious, totally accepted, full of hope and love, and that we have a wonderful future ahead? What might be possible? **Once we discover our true value, it's so much easier to stay motivated to attain and maintain real, authentic healing and wellness.**

No matter what you've been told or have experienced, you are so loved. *God really does love you . . . and He is good!* He made you a one-of-a-kind original for His plan of peace, prosperity, and hope for your life. He's not looking for performance. He's not waiting to zap you, and He's not mad at you. Quite the opposite. Only with Him will you be fully satisfied, be good enough, and find true value, hope, and meaning for life. Without these vital answers and keys to living, we aimlessly and futilely attempt to soothe and fill these needs with something else. Often, it's food. But, **it is only Love that completely heals**.

You can only truly experience radiant living by joining your life to Love . . . the One who sees you as perfect and priceless, the One who knows your beginning, your end, and every day in-between. He alone can break the chains of life's pain, traumas, frustrations, shame, and guilt, wiping the slate clean and **giving you**

a brand-new start. He alone wants to share His perfection and beauty with you, giving you real, unrivaled value, and purpose. Then, you can step past the barriers, get to know this Perfect Love, and move into His incredible plan for your life that He designed long before you even existed.

The Love of God alone can heal every area of your life—body, mind, and spirit—completely. In fact, that's just who He is: Restorer. Because of the mercy, compassion, and kindness of our God, His Light shines upon us when we sit huddled in shadowy places of darkness and death. The Light helps us rise up and walk, one step at a time, guiding our feet onto pathways of peace.

So let the Light shine into those dark places, the places that taunt, intimidate, obscure, and distort your value and future. **Let it bring supernatural healing, forgiveness, joy and restoration to those hidden and broken places of trauma, pain, grief, and shame in your heart.** God loves *you*. *You* have purpose. *You* have value. *You* have a destiny that's ready to be fulfilled. And *many* are waiting and depending on what *only you* can bring. Know that you are worth the investment. And get ready for the exciting future that lies ahead.

Love is calling you. Will you receive the gift?

My heart and hope is for you to personally experience as I have, this same Love, Power, and Healing that transforms darkness to light, death to life, and ashes to beauty. As our journey together in these pages is nearing an end, I want to leave you with a blessing of healing and hope and one that will introduce you to real Love:

Dearest Love and Father, I pray that You bless Your dear Princess or Prince now with a long, fulfilling and healthy life. Make Yourself so real to them. Shower them with Your Love, Your Forgiveness, Your Healing, Your Freedom, and Your Peace. Help them see and accept that each of us has messed up royally and all our attempts to attain a life equal to God's perfection have failed and are useless. Though the payoff for a life separated from You is death, instead, You took that for us and offer a *totally free gift of real life*, forever life through Jesus to anyone who calls out to You. Meet the one calling to You now. Wash them, change them, set them free and make them completely brand new. Fill them with Your Spirit of Resurrection Life. Lead them out of the stuck places and the pain in their lives and guide them into all of the peace, purpose, destiny, and life You have planned for them, in Jesus Mighty and Precious Name.

If you're experiencing pain or illness in your body, I release the Healing Presence, Power, and Love of the Kingdom of Heaven to come upon you now. I command Healing and Life to flood your body, heart, and mind. All pain, disease, and sickness must leave. All grief and heaviness must go. I speak joy and peace to you—body, mind, and spirit. Peace. Peace…in Jesus Name.

No matter where you are on your journey, be inspired to keep going. Don't give up. Let weariness fall away. Step in more deeply. There is so much more. This is still just the beginning. Dive in and let Love overtake every part of you. **Taste and see how *good* it is.** Peace, joy, freedom, purpose, fulfillment, and radiance are ahead as you walk out this journey of Love and real, sweet health and wellness.

Recipes

Here are a few favorites that came out of my food adventures and continue to keep the path doable, satisfying, and flavorful for me and my family. Now it's your turn to indulge . . . innocently!

Desserts

Innocent Indulgence –
Lemon Island Cheesecake

Innocent Indulgence –
Fudge Brownies

Cookie Dough

Creamy Banana Soft Serve

Innocent Indulgence –
Chocolate Fudge

Every Day Is a Holiday

Guacamole

Grandma's Favorite Cranberries

Sweet Potato Fries

Morning Starters

Oat Granola

Lemon Chia Seed Muffins

Smoothies

Spiced Pear-Apple Smoothie

Anytime Green Smoothie

Peanut Butter-Banana Shake

Soups

Split Pea Soup

Veggie Chili

Bean and Kale Stew

Salads

Spring Roll Salad

Mediterranean Kale Salad

Pomegranate and Greens

Modern Favorites

Italian Zucchini Melt

Easy Spaghetti

Fish Taco Wraps

DESSERTS

INNOCENT INDULGENCE – LEMON ISLAND CHEESECAKE

Filling

2⅔ cups raw cashews, sorted
½ cup coconut oil
1⅓ cups lemon juice, with pulp
Zest from 1 medium lemon
2 teaspoons vanilla
⅔ cup raw honey (or to taste depending on sourness of lemons)
¼ teaspoon KAL® Pure Stevia Extract (powder)
⅛ teaspoon sea salt
½ cup shredded coconut (unsweetened)

1. Soak cashews, covering with 2-inches of water. Cover with a lid, then refrigerate overnight.
2. The next day, rinse and drain the cashews. Trim away any dark spots or blemishes on the nuts, and set aside.
3. Seasonal note: If cold, gently warm the coconut oil and honey to soften.
4. Blend coconut oil, lemon juice, zest, vanilla, honey, stevia, and sea salt in a high-powered blender.
5. Gradually add in soaked cashews, processing and stirring until smooth and creamy.
6. Add shredded coconut and continue to blend on high to desired texture.

Crust

⅔ cup almond meal
¼ teaspoon sea salt
⅔ cup raw macadamia nuts
1½ tablespoons raw honey
½ cup medjool dates, chopped
½ cup shredded coconut (unsweetened)

1. Blend almond meal and sea salt on high in food processor to form a fine powder.
2. Add macadamia nuts, and pulse process until well-chopped and just starting to stick together, being careful not to over-process the mixture into an oily paste.
3. Process in dates until mixed.
4. Process in coconut until just chopped.
5. Pulse to mix in honey.
6. Grease or line one 8- or 9-inch (or four 4-inch) spring-form pan(s) with parchment paper. OR, use a muffin pan to make 12 individual cheesecakes. Firmly, press in crust to desired, uniform thickness. Pour in filling, spreading evenly, then freeze. Extra crust can be shaped into delicious cookies.

To serve: Thaw until partially frozen and slice with a large knife, wiping blade clean between cuts. Plate and enjoy while still slightly frozen or well-chilled. Freeze or refrigerate any remaining portions.

Makes: 12 servings

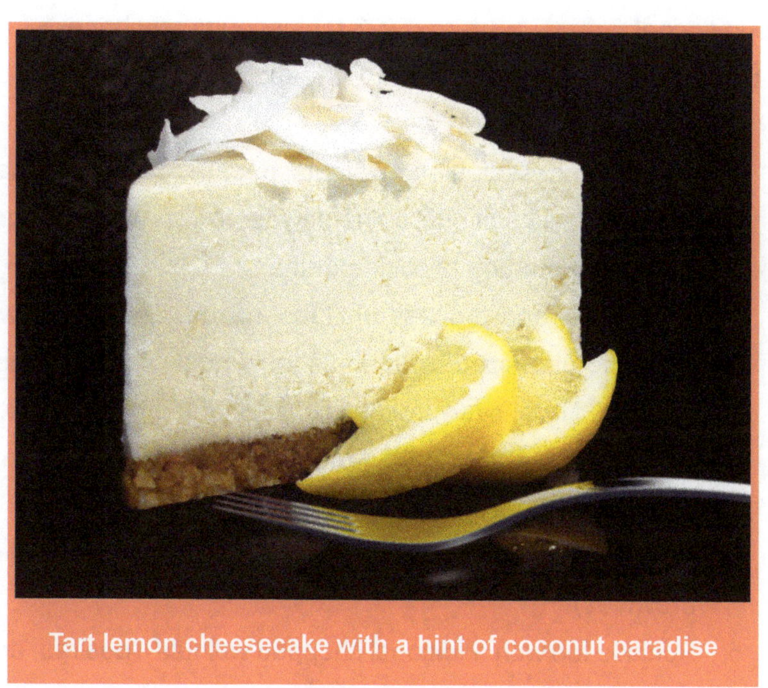

Tart lemon cheesecake with a hint of coconut paradise

INNOCENT INDULGENCE – FUDGE BROWNIES

1¼ cups pecans
1¼ cups walnuts
1 cup cocoa*
¼ teaspoon sea salt
¼ teaspoon xanthan gum
½ cup dates, finely chopped
3 tablespoons raw honey
1½ teaspoons vanilla

1. In food processor, blend walnuts, pecans, cocoa, xanthan gum, and sea salt until a fine powder forms, with the ingredients just starting to stick together.
2. Add dates, and process until just mixed. The dough will form into pea-sized balls and should hold its shape when pinched. Note: over-processing will make oily brownies.
3. Add honey and vanilla, and pulse-chop on low until just mixed.
4. Press into an 8-inch square pan (or smaller for thicker brownies).
5. Sprinkle top with additional chopped walnuts if desired, and lightly press to keep in place.

*100 percent dark cocoa powder, not Dutch chocolate or processed with alkali

Makes: 12-16 brownies

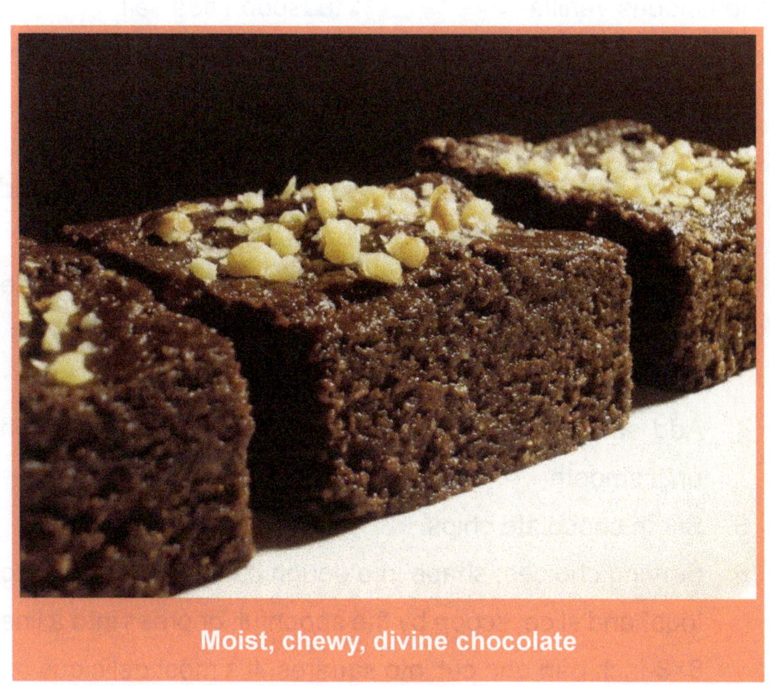

Moist, chewy, divine chocolate

COOKIE DOUGH

1 can (15 oz.) garbanzo beans, rinsed and drained well
4 large dates, pitted and minced
⅓ cup cashew butter
2¾ teaspoons vanilla
½ cup brown coconut sugar
½ cup multi-blend gluten-free flour (high fiber, if possible)
2 tablespoons xylitol
½ teaspoon baking soda
¼ teaspoon sea salt
⅔ cup semi-sweet chocolate chips or chunks*

1. Grind beans in an 11- to 14-cup food processor. (Divide into batches if using a smaller size.)
2. Add minced dates, and process again until very well blended.
3. Blend in cashew butter and vanilla, processing to form a smooth paste.
4. Add all combined dry ingredients, stirring and blending until smooth.
5. Stir in chocolate chips.
6. Serving choices: shape into dough balls, form into "dough logs" and slice, scoop by the spoonful, or press into a lined 8×8-inch pan and cut into squares. It's most delicious and easiest to cut well-chilled. Do not bake.
7. Store in the freezer (if it lasts that long), as dough thaws quickly.

*Options: Try stevia-sweetened chips, or chop a xylitol-sweetened dark chocolate bar.

Makes: 24 dough balls or 4 – 1×6-inch dough logs

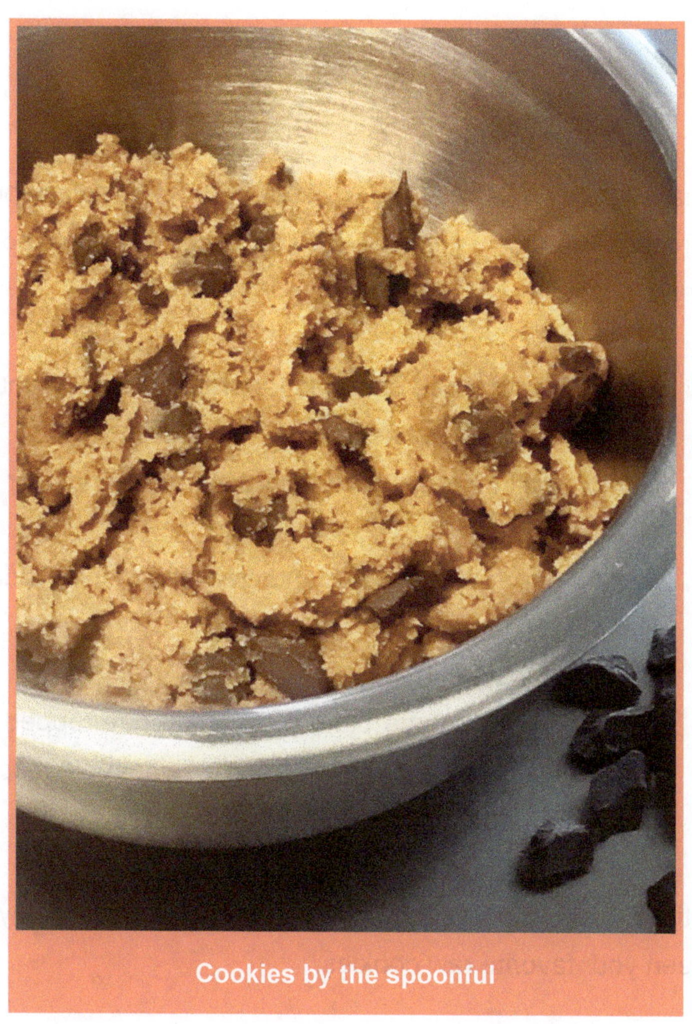

Cookies by the spoonful

CREAMY BANANA SOFT SERVE

4 bananas, peeled, sliced, and frozen
1 teaspoon vanilla
2½ tablespoons cashew butter
2½ tablespoons lucuma powder

1. Partially thaw sliced bananas (approximately 10 minutes) to make blending easier.
2. Combine all ingredients in high-powered blender or food processor.
3. Blend on high until smooth and creamy, scraping sides of blender as needed.
4. Serve immediately.
5. Enjoy your soft serve plain or as a sundae topped with cocoa nibs, berries, chopped pecans, pineapple, coconut, and chocolate fudge, or layered as a parfait.

Variations: Make cookie sandwiches by freezing soft serve layered between your favorite raw cookies.

Makes: 4-5 servings (½ cup)

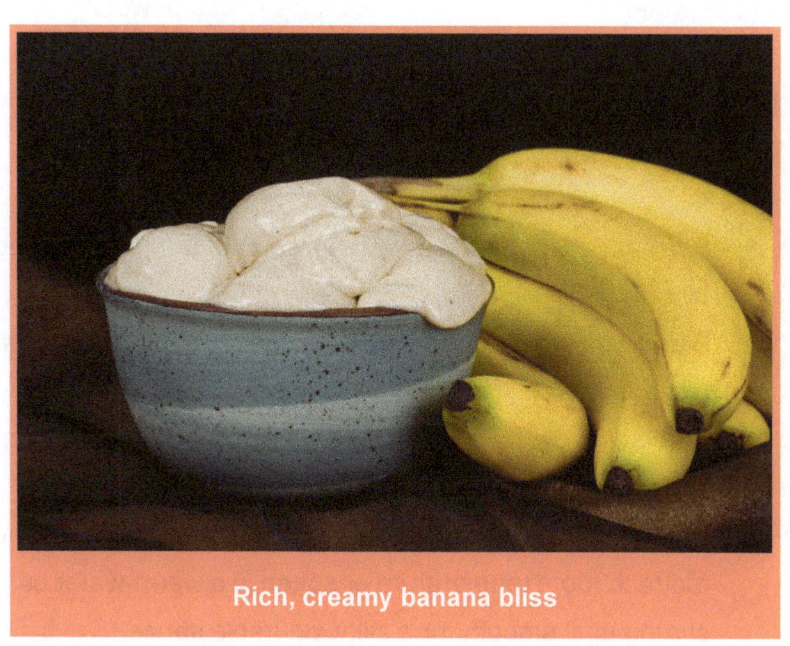

Rich, creamy banana bliss

INNOCENT INDULGENCE – CHOCOLATE FUDGE

1½ cups water
½ cup raw honey
3 tablespoons coconut oil
2¼ teaspoons vanilla
2¾ cups cocoa powder*
½ teaspoon KAL® Pure Stevia Extract (powder)

1. For easy mixing, place wet ingredients in high-powered blender first, then add dry ingredients.
2. Blend on high until smooth and creamy, stirring occasionally to mix well.
3. Serve as a dip for fresh fruit, scoop on nondairy ice cream, or just enjoy by the spoonful.
4. Refrigerate or freeze remaining portions. Bring chilled fudge to room temperature or soften in a warm-water bath, stirring until smooth for a silky, pourable sauce.

*100 percent dark cocoa powder, not Dutch chocolate or processed with alkali

Makes: 24 servings (2 tablespoons)

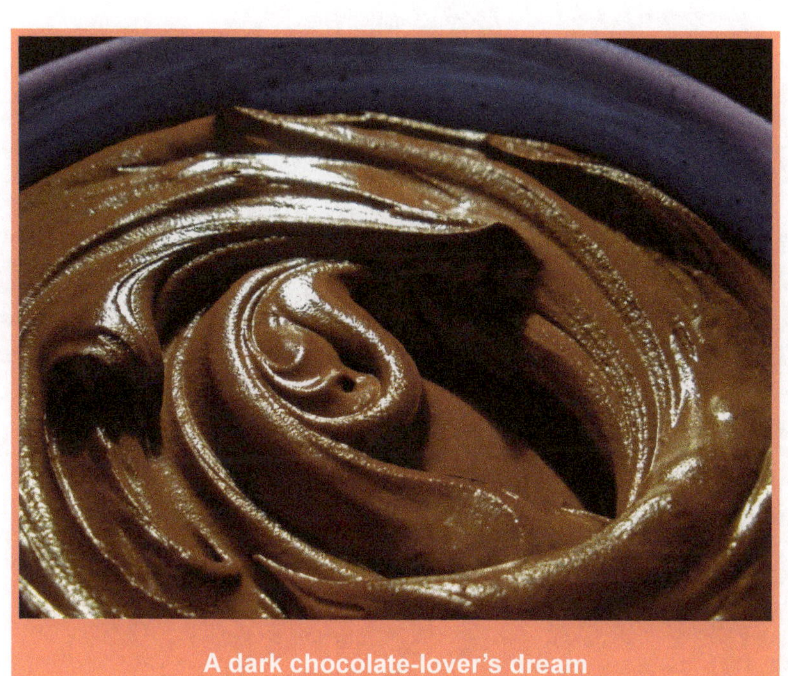

A dark chocolate-lover's dream

EVERY DAY IS A HOLIDAY

GUACAMOLE

3 avocados, mashed chunkily with a fork
3 Roma tomatoes, chopped
2 garlic cloves, minced
2 teaspoons lime or lemon juice
½ teaspoon sea salt
⅔ cup chopped red or sweet onion

1. Stir just to combine all ingredients in small bowl. Serve immediately.
2. Refrigerate remaining portions in an airtight container, including one of the pits to keep color fresh.

Serving suggestions:

- Dip with jicama, veggies, baked corn chips, and/or flax crackers
- Fill mushroom caps
- Spread on burritos or wraps
- Dollop on salads, tostadas, or tacos

Makes: 4-6 servings (½ cup)

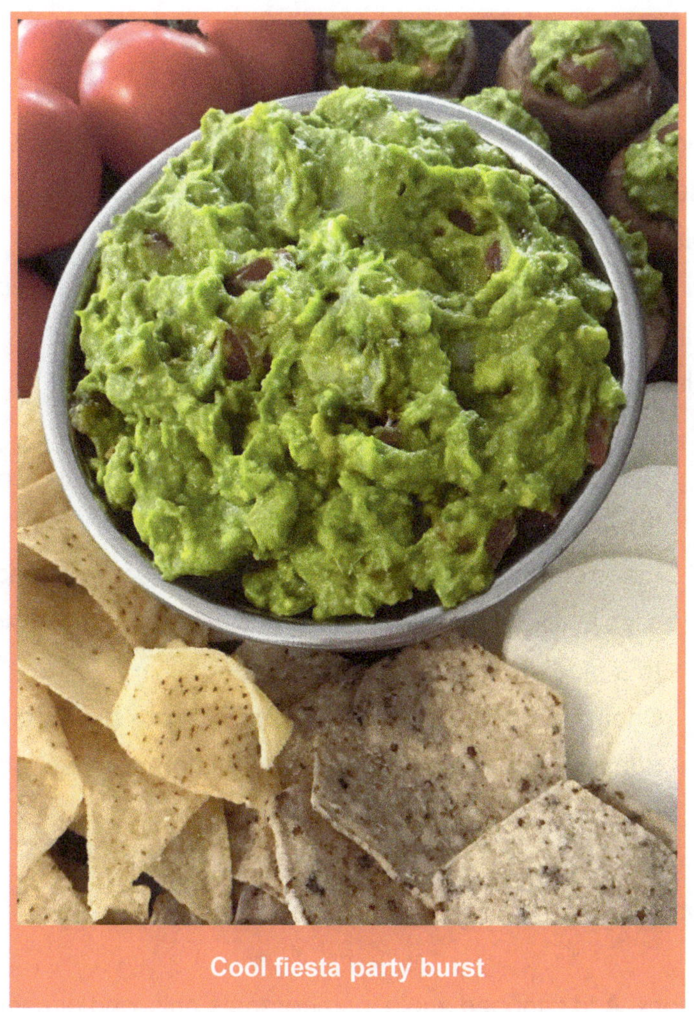

Cool fiesta party burst

GRANDMA'S FAVORITE CRANBERRIES

2 medium oranges with peel, washed and quartered
3 tablespoons raw honey, softened slightly in a warm-water bath if needed
2 tablespoons xylitol
2 scoops KAL® Pure Stevia Extract (powder)*
4½ cups fresh or frozen cranberries, rinsed and drained

1. Remove orange seeds, stems, and half of the orange peels, leaving the remaining peels intact.
2. Place oranges and sweeteners in food processor, and process until slightly chunky, but peel is well chopped. Transfer to a medium-sized mixing bowl.
3. Chop cranberries in food processor, leaving slightly chunky.
4. Stir together sweetened oranges and cranberries, adding additional sweetener if needed.

*Scoop comes in jar

Variations: Add chopped apple, pomegranate arils, and/or chopped nuts (walnuts, pecans).

Makes: 12-16 servings (¼ cup)

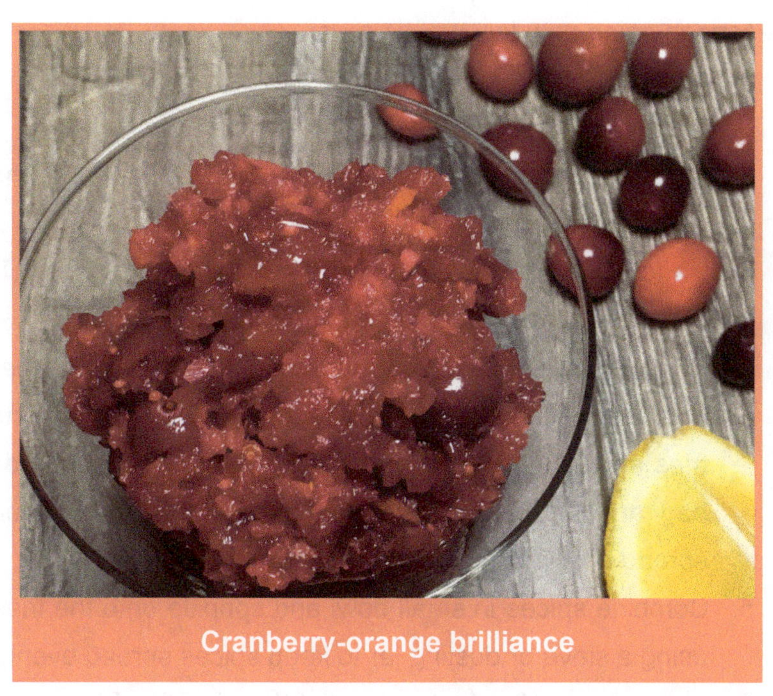

Cranberry-orange brilliance

SWEET POTATO FRIES

4 medium sweet potatoes
1 teaspoon garlic powder
2 teaspoons chili powder
1 teaspoon onion powder
Cayenne, to taste
½ teaspoon sea salt
Olive oil spray

1. Preheat oven to 450°F.
2. Wash and dry sweet potatoes. Trim out "eyes" and dark spots.
3. Uniformly slice sweet potatoes into long strips or circle-shaped fries (or waffle cut).
4. Place on a foil-covered or parchment-lined baking sheet. Mist/spray both sides of fries with olive oil. (OR, add cut fries and 2-3 tablespoons olive oil to gallon-sized Ziploc bag and shake/mix/massage to coat potatoes. Then spread onto baking sheet.)
5. Combine spices in small bowl and sprinkle onto the fries, using a sieve or dusting jar to keep spices spread evenly.
6. Bake about 10 minutes to slightly crisp the fries, then stir and flip.
7. Bake another 10–15 minutes until fries are crispy but tender.
8. Enjoy plain or with ketchup.

Makes: 4 servings

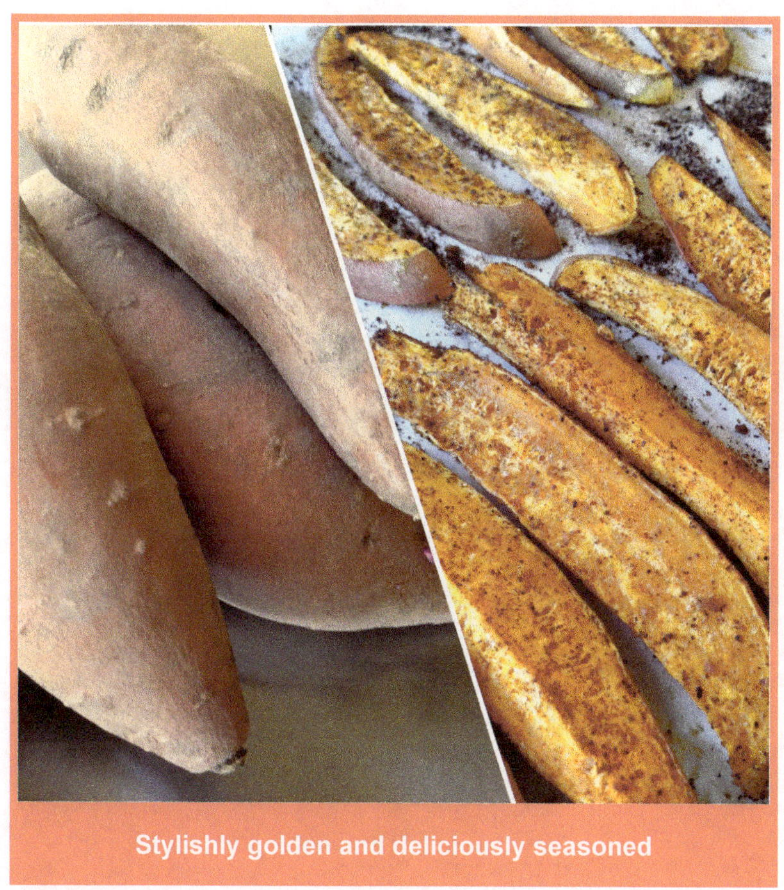

Stylishly golden and deliciously seasoned

MORNING STARTERS

OAT GRANOLA

3 cups old-fashioned oats (regular or gluten-free)
½ cup chopped nuts or seeds (walnuts, almonds, pecans, pumpkin seeds)
½ cup ground flaxseed*
½ cup unsweetened coconut
1¾ teaspoons cinnamon (optional)
⅛ teaspoon sea salt
3 tablespoons xylitol**

1. In a medium mixing bowl or 2-quart storage container, mix (or shake) together all ingredients.
2. Serve with your favorite fresh fruit (blueberries, blackberries, raspberries, cherries, peaches, apples, bananas) and/or dried fruit (raisins, cranberries), and a milk alternative.
3. Store refrigerated in an airtight container.

*Or chia seed, but add to individual servings

**Or sweeten with your favorite natural sweetener

Makes: 8 servings (½ cup)

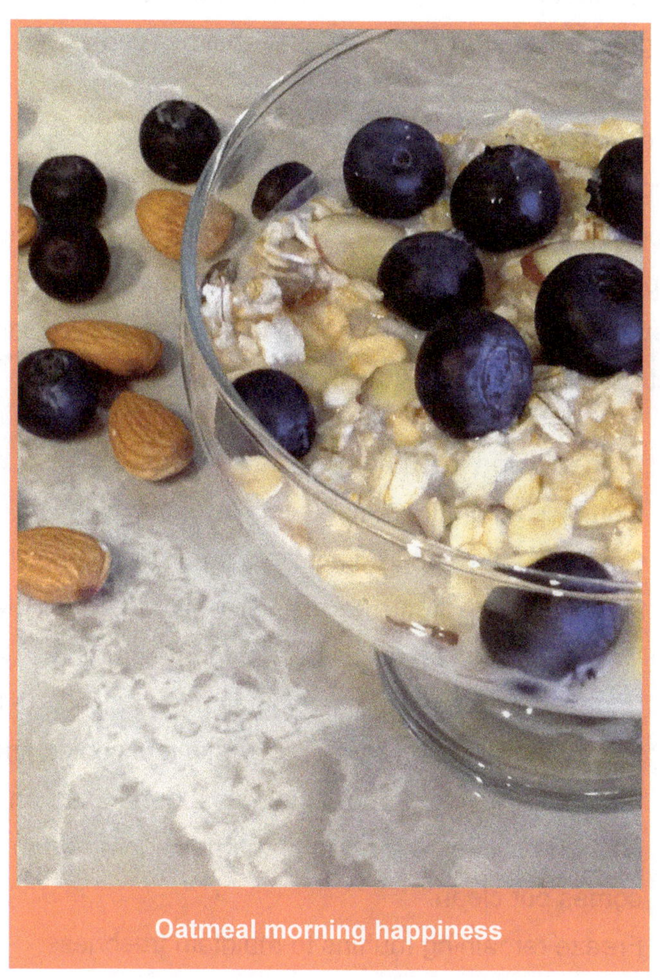
Oatmeal morning happiness

LEMON CHIA SEED MUFFINS

1½ cups gluten-free flour blend*
¾ cup coconut flour
⅔ cup ground flaxseed
⅓ cup xylitol
¼ cup chia seeds
½ teaspoon sea salt
1 teaspoon baking soda
5 teaspoons baking powder
¼ teaspoon KAL® Pure Stevia Extract (powder)
¼ teaspoon xanthan gum
2 tablespoons raw honey (soften if needed)
¼ cup coconut oil (soften if needed)
1 cup lemon juice
Zest from 1 medium lemon
2 teaspoons vanilla
1¼ teaspoons lemon extract
2 eggs, beaten

1. Preheat oven to 350°F.
2. Combine all dry ingredients in a large mixing bowl.
3. Combine all wet ingredients in a small mixing bowl.
4. Add wet ingredients to dry, and stir until just blended. Dough will thicken quickly and become crumbly.
5. Scoop into greased or lined muffin pan, making 10-12 muffins. (I like silicon pans on stainless steel cookie sheets.)
6. Bake at 350°F for 25 to 30 minutes, depending on muffin size and pan type, and until toothpick inserted in center comes out clean.
7. Freeze remaining muffins to maintain freshness.

*Arrowhead Mills® Gluten Free All-Purpose Flour gave the best results.

Makes: 10-12 muffins

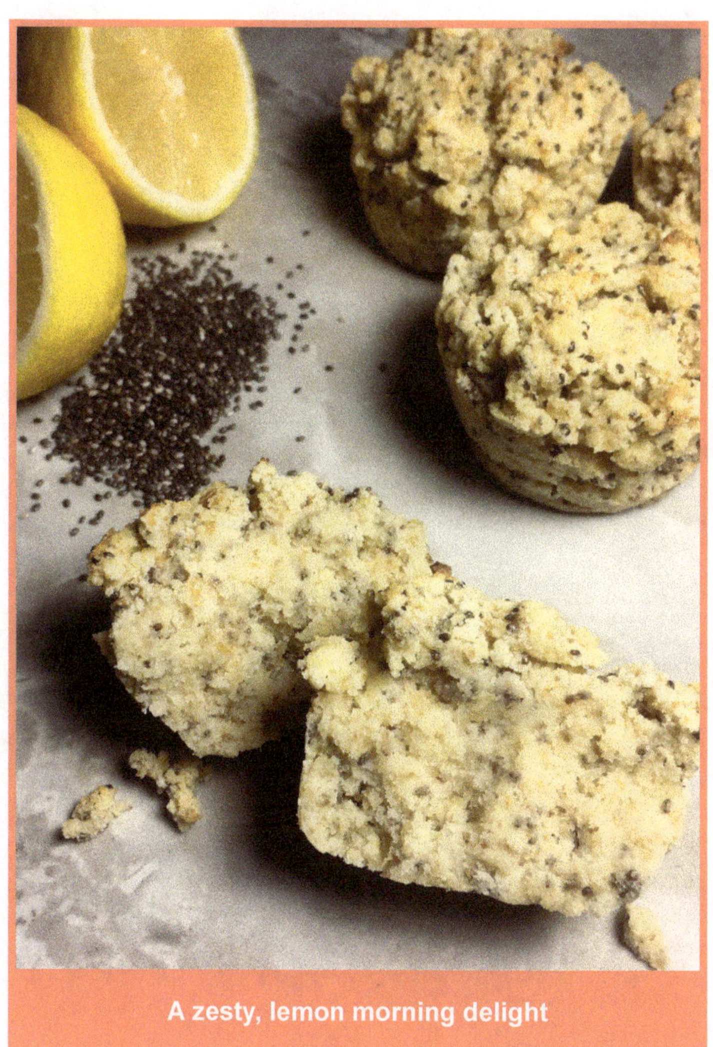

A zesty, lemon morning delight

SMOOTHIES

SPICED PEAR-APPLE SMOOTHIE

2 medium Bartlett pears, quartered and frozen
1 medium banana
1 Granny Smith apple, cored
1 Medjool date, pitted (or 1 tablespoon brown coconut sugar)
16 pecan halves
⅓ cup vanilla almond milk, unsweetened
1-2 tablespoons flaxseed oil, optional
1-2 tablespoons chia seed or flaxseed, optional
1 tablespoon lemon juice
¼ teaspoon cinnamon
¾ teaspoon vanilla
1 scoop KAL® Pure Stevia Extract (powder)*
2 servings protein powder, optional**
2 cups ice cubes

1. Load liquids and soft fruits in high-powered blender first and frozen ingredients last.
2. Blend all ingredients until smooth.

*Scoop comes in jar

**Measure servings according to package instructions. Whey from grass-fed cows and plant-based, raw protein meal blends are my favorites. Different types may alter the flavor and may require more or less sweetener or liquid to be used in the smoothie.

Makes: approximately 3 servings (12 oz.)

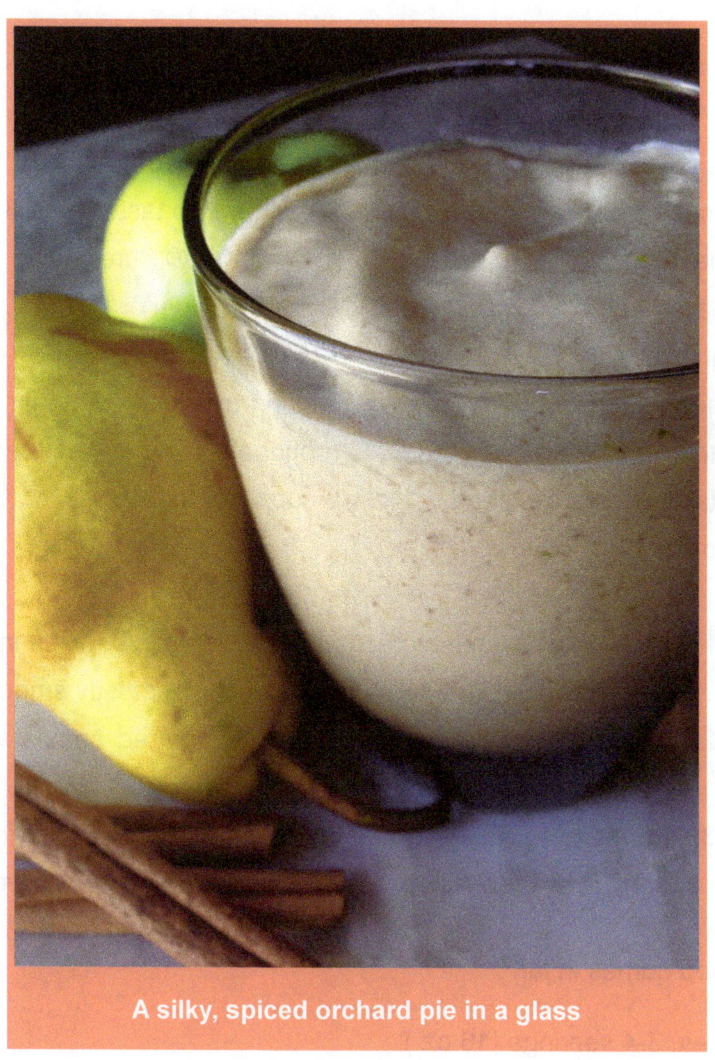

A silky, spiced orchard pie in a glass

ANYTIME GREEN SMOOTHIE

½ lb. spinach, washed and dried

1¼ cups fresh or frozen pineapple chunks

1 pear or apple, cored

1 banana

1 lime, peeled

2 cups cold water

1-2 tablespoons flaxseed oil, optional

¼-⅓ cup chia or flax seed

Sweetener to taste (I like 3 scoops KAL® Pure Stevia Extract powder)*

1 teaspoon ground ginger, or 1-inch fresh, peeled ginger (optional)

2 cups ice, to taste

1. Starting with liquids, pack all ingredients except ice into a high-powered blender, and process until mostly smooth.
2. Add ice and continue blending to desired consistency. Serve immediately.
3. For easy mornings, make the night before and store in airtight glass jar(s), filled to the top. (Canning jars work great.)

*Scoop comes in jar

Makes: 3-4 servings (16 oz.)

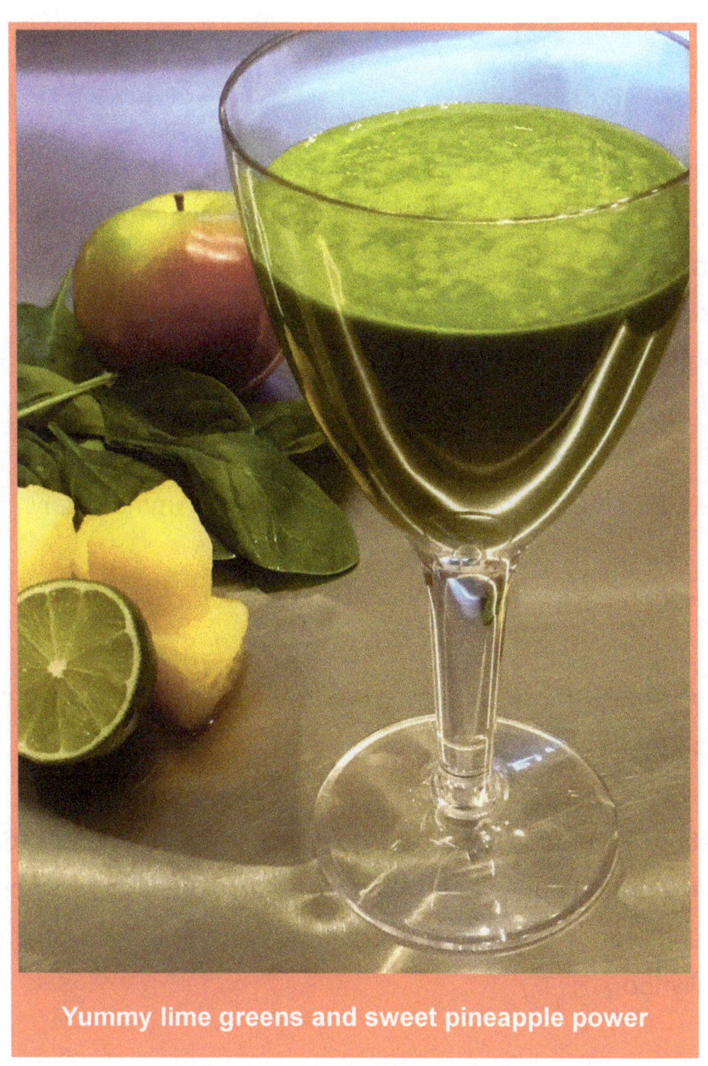

Yummy lime greens and sweet pineapple power

PEANUT BUTTER-BANANA SHAKE

1 banana, chilled or frozen
2 tablespoons peanut butter*
½ teaspoon vanilla
1 cup ice
Cinnamon, to taste
Sea salt, pinch
Protein powder (optional)**
½ cup vanilla almond milk, unsweetened

1. Load blender, starting with liquid ingredients first.
2. Blend until smooth and creamy. Serve immediately.

*Any nut butter works

**May require more or less sweetener, depending on protein being used

Variation: Peanut butter always goes with chocolate, so try adding 1½ tablespoons unsweetened cocoa and honey or another natural sweetener to taste. Chocolate protein powder works wonderfully too.

Makes: 1 serving (16 oz.)

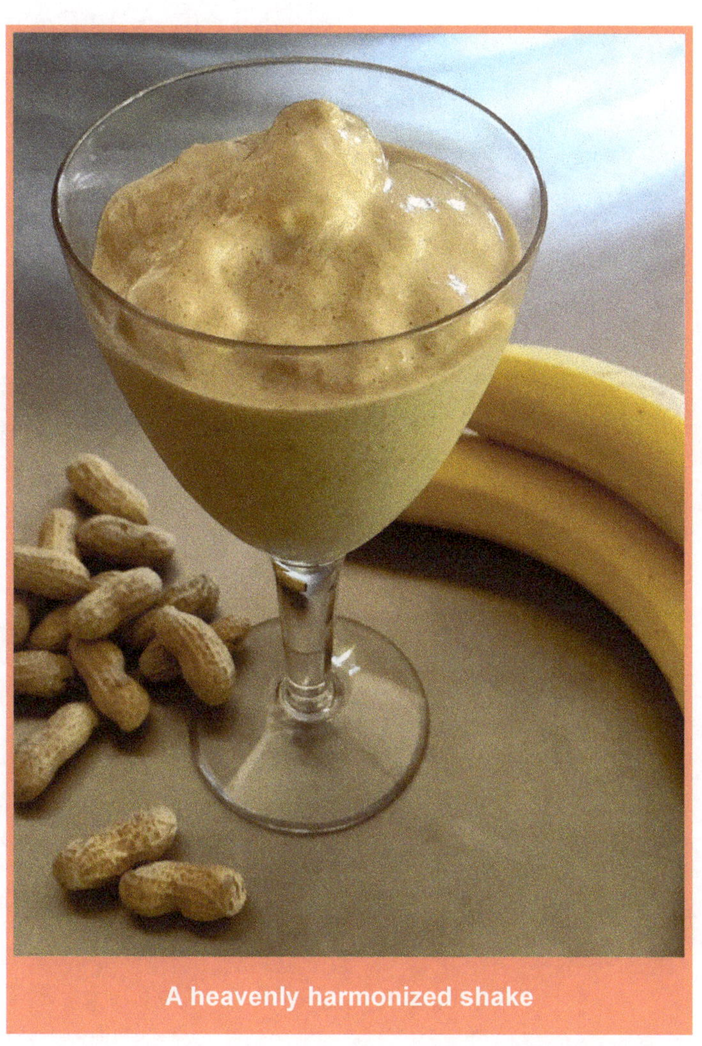

A heavenly harmonized shake

SOUPS

SPLIT PEA SOUP

1¾ lbs. dry green split peas (no overnight soaking required)
3 qts. water
3 medium carrots, diced
1½ stalks celery, diced
½ onion, diced
2 garlic cloves, minced
1 medium red potato with skin, diced (rinse and drain to reduce starch if desired)
¼ teaspoon black pepper
2-2¼ teaspoons sea salt*

1. Check peas carefully for stones and bad peas, and remove. Wash and drain peas. Place peas in a 6-quart pot (or larger) with water, and bring to a boil. Simmer uncovered for 2 minutes. (Caution: This easily boils over.)
2. Add veggies and simmer partially covered, until veggies are soft and peas reach desired consistency. Stir occasionally (a spatula works best), and adjust the temperature as needed to prevent sticking or boiling-over. Cook about 2 hours.
3. Stir in salt to taste, and serve.
4. Refrigerate or freeze remaining portions. Add small amount of water when reheating, as soup thickens after being chilled.

*Be sure to add salt after soup is finished. Adding salt too early will prevent peas from softening.

Makes: 9-10 servings (1½ cups)

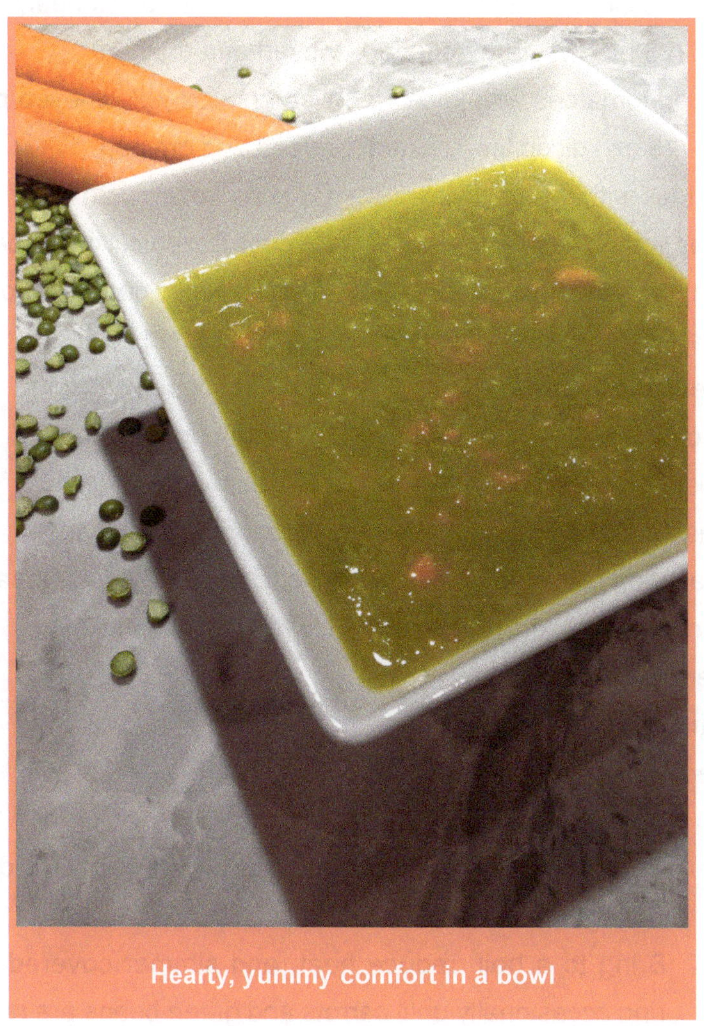

Hearty, yummy comfort in a bowl

VEGGIE CHILI

2-4 garlic cloves, minced
1 can (28 oz.) whole (chopped) or diced tomatoes with juice
1 can (15 oz.) diced fire-roasted tomatoes with green chilies
3 cups water
1 can (6 oz.) tomato paste
2-3 tablespoons chili powder
1½ teaspoons powdered mustard
1 teaspoon dried basil
1 teaspoon dried oregano
½ teaspoon ground cumin
1 can (15 oz.) kidney beans, rinsed and drained
1 can (15 oz.) garbanzo beans, rinsed and drained
1 can (15 oz.) black beans, rinsed and drained
1 can (15 oz.) black-eyed peas, rinsed and drained
1½ cups frozen corn
1½ cups frozen cut green beans
1½ cups sliced carrots (about 3)
½ cup chopped celery
2 cups chopped zucchini
1 medium onion, chopped
1½ teaspoons sea salt
½ teaspoon black pepper
½ cup seafood cocktail sauce, low-sugar (optional)

1. Combine all ingredients in a large soup pot (6-quart or larger).
2. Bring to a boil, reduce heat, and simmer covered, stirring occasionally until carrots and green beans are tender, about 15-20 minutes.

Makes: 10-11 servings (1½ cups)

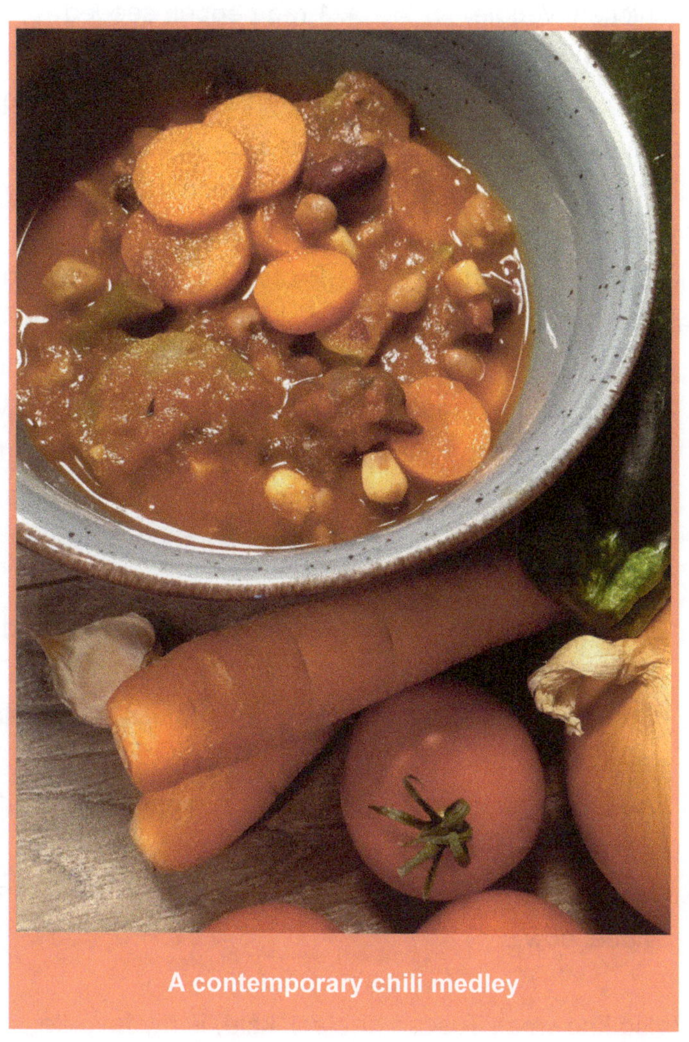

A contemporary chili medley

BEAN AND KALE STEW

4 cups water
2 cups low-sodium broth (chicken, veggie, or mushroom)
4 cans (15 oz.) great northern beans, rinsed, drained, and divided
1 tablespoon olive oil
2 garlic cloves, minced
1 small onion, chopped
½ cup chopped celery
1½ cups chopped carrots
1 red pepper, seeded and chopped
1 lb. kale, deveined and chopped*
½ teaspoon sea salt
¼ teaspoon freshly ground black pepper
Protein of choice, precooked (optional)**

1. In 6-quart pot, sauté garlic, onion, and celery in olive oil. Add water, broth, and 2 cans of whole great northern beans. Bring to a boil as you prep the other veggies. (For a shortcut, skip sautéing and just combine all seven ingredients in soup pot.)
2. Fork-mash the remaining 2 cans of beans, and add to the stew.
3. Stir in remaining veggies and seasonings, continuing to heat to a boil.
4. Reduce heat, partially cover, and simmer for about 15-20 minutes, until carrots and kale soften.
5. Mix in your protein just before serving, or garnish individual bowls.

*Dino (also known as Tuscan or black kale) is my favorite.
**Try crispy, turkey bacon crumbles or lean, ground, white turkey breast.

Makes: 8 servings (1½ cups)

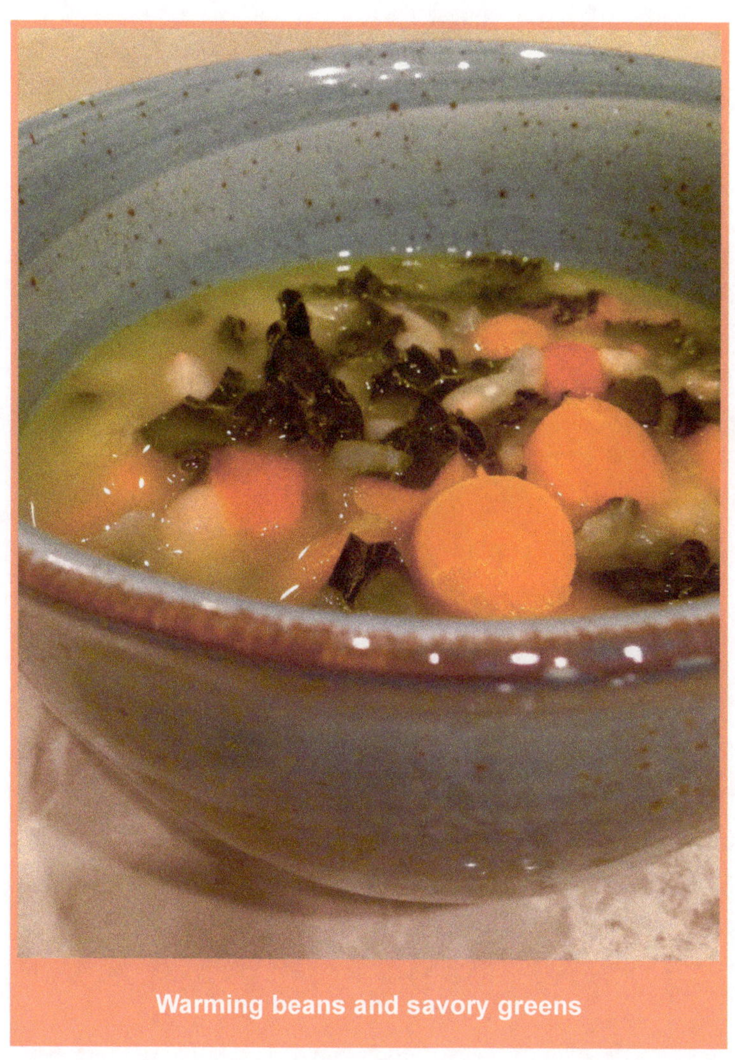

Warming beans and savory greens

SALADS

SPRING ROLL SALAD

Salad

½ head green cabbage, shredded or chopped
½ head purple cabbage, shredded or chopped
1 red pepper, chopped
1 sweet onion, chopped
4 carrots, shredded or chopped
6-8 mushrooms, sliced
1½ cups mango, chopped
½-⅔ cup raw cashews, chopped
1-2 avocados, sliced
1 handful fresh cilantro, roughly chopped
1 handful fresh basil, julienned
Red pepper flakes, optional

Dressing

¼ cup coconut aminos* or low-sodium tamari
2 tablespoons raw honey*
1½ teaspoons sesame oil
¼ cup water
1¼ teaspoons dried ginger*
1 clove garlic, minced

1. Make dressing first to allow flavors to mingle. Combine all ingredients in blender, processing until smooth.
2. For salad, toss all ingredients together in a large bowl.
3. Serve dressing on the side or pour desired amount over salad and toss.
4. Garnish with red pepper flakes, if desired.

*If using coconut aminos instead of tamari, increase aminos to ½ cup and reduce honey to 1½-2 teaspoons and ginger to ¾-1 teaspoon.

Makes: 6 large salads

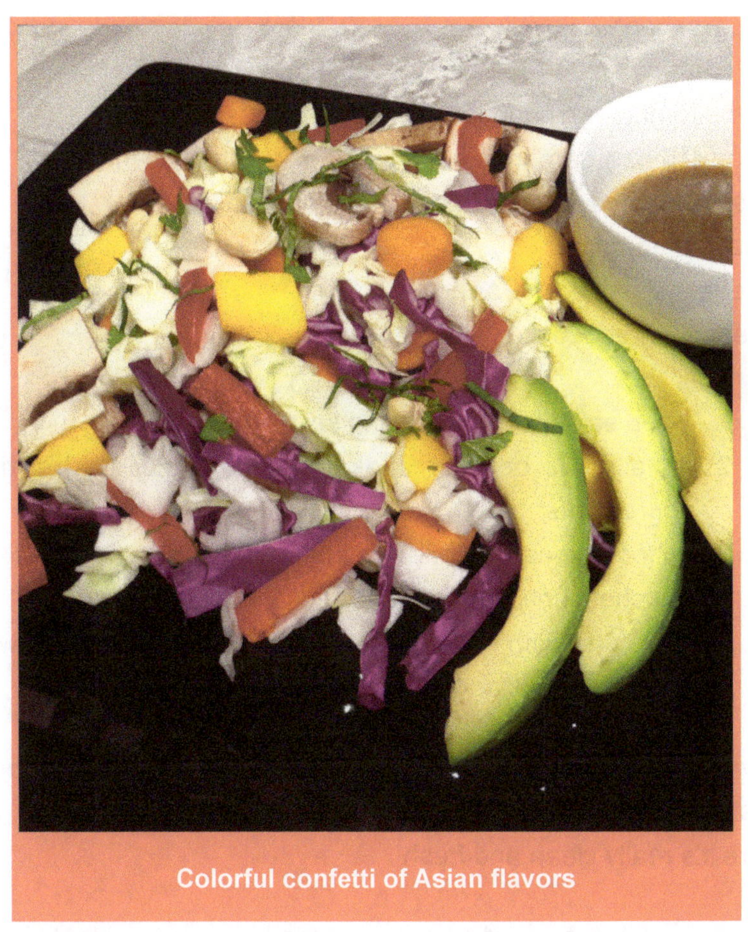

Colorful confetti of Asian flavors

MEDITERRANEAN KALE SALAD

Salad

2 bunches dino kale, deveined and washed*
3 Roma tomatoes (or 1 cup grape tomatoes), chopped
1 can (15 oz.) garbanzo beans, rinsed, drained, and heated
Sea salt, to taste
Avocado, sliced or Parmesan cheese, shredded

Dressing

2 lemons, juiced (about ⅓ cup)
2-4 large garlic cloves, minced
⅓ cup extra virgin olive oil, cold pressed
Sea salt and cayenne pepper, to taste

1. Prep salad ingredients and set aside.
2. In a small bowl or shaker jar, combine all dressing ingredients.
3. In food processor, pulse-chop kale and dressing in divided batches, until kale is bite-sized. Stir to combine.**
4. Top salad with tomatoes and warm beans, garnishing with Parmesan or avocado, as desired.

*Dino (also known as Tuscan and black kale) is a milder variety. Make prep easy by using 2 bags washed and chopped kale. Be sure it's really clean and fresh!

**To make without a food processor: chop kale and transfer to large salad bowl. Sprinkle with sea salt and hand-squeeze/massage chopped leaves for a couple of minutes to soften the greens. Pour on dressing and toss.

Makes: 3 large salads

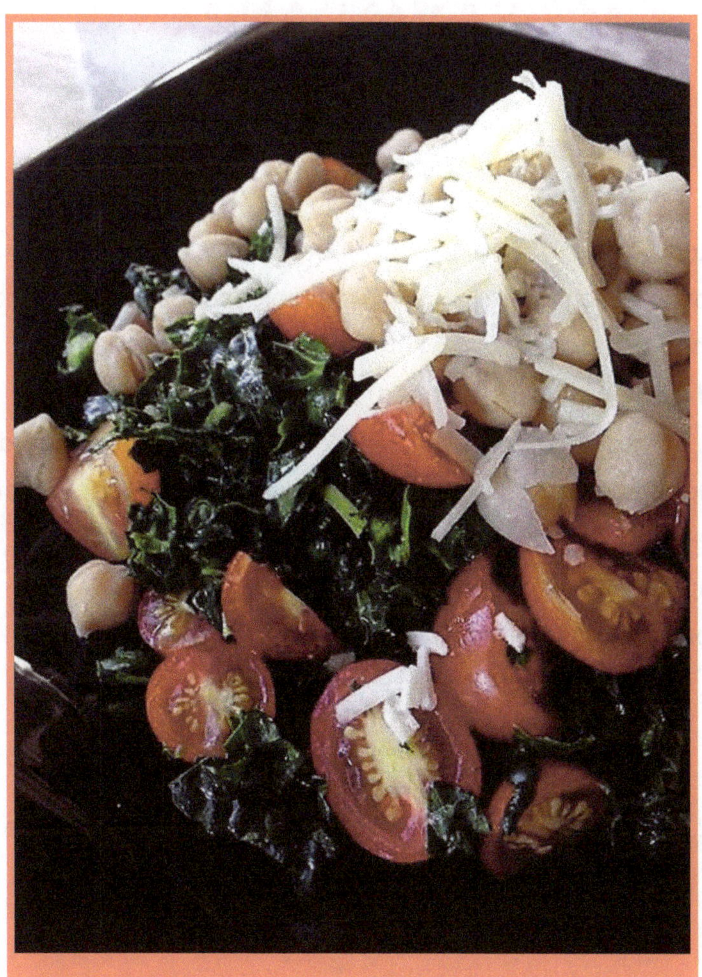

Robustly delicious, garlicky kale and bright tomatoes

POMEGRANATE AND GREENS

Salad

5-8 oz. spinach, washed and dried

1 red apple with skin, chopped

8 oz. pomegranate arils

½ cup dried cherries (fruit-juice sweetened), chopped

½ cup pecans, chopped

4-6 oz. feta, crumbled (I like goat or sheep)

Dressing

6 tablespoons coconut vinegar

6 tablespoons olive oil

3 tablespoons raw honey

2 teaspoons spicy mustard

Sea salt and pepper to taste

1. Layer salad in bowl(s).
2. In shaker jar, combine dressing ingredients and shake until blended. Serve on the side or pour desired amount over salad, and toss.

Makes: 3-4 servings (3 cups)

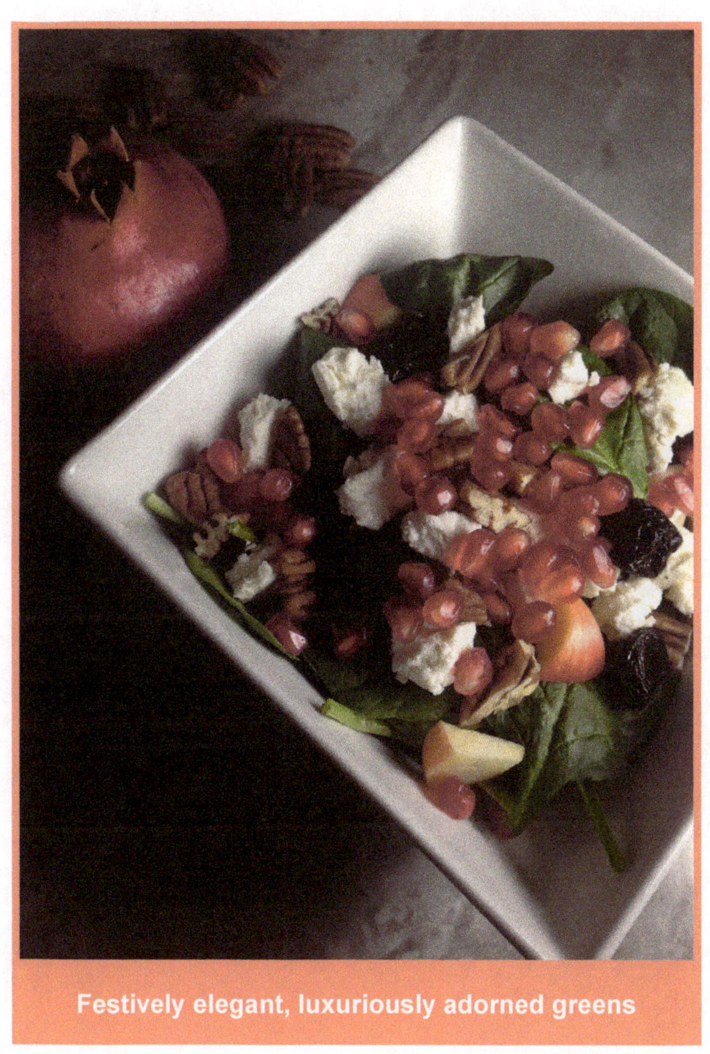

Festively elegant, luxuriously adorned greens

MODERN FAVORITES

ITALIAN ZUCCHINI MELT

3 zucchinis, washed and thinly sliced (pieces, ribbons or spiralized)
4-6 mushrooms, sliced
½-¾ sweet onion, chopped
½-¾ green pepper, chopped
3-6 Roma tomatoes (or the equivalent in grape tomatoes), chopped
Your choice of protein (e.g., ground turkey, lean ground beef, uncured turkey pepperoni), hot/warmed
1 can (15 oz.) garbanzo beans, rinsed, drained, and heated
1-1½ cups organic shredded mozzarella or parmesan cheese
Italian seasoning or fresh basil

1. Lightly sauté onions and peppers. Add mushrooms and continue to sauté, just to soften but retain veggies' crispness; set aside.
2. Stir-fry zucchini and layer in bottom of individual-serving, oven-proof dishes.*
3. Top with sautéed mushrooms, onions, peppers, beans, tomatoes, and your choice of protein and/or cheese.
4. Warm and melt in 350°F oven about 5 minutes, just until cheese is bubbly.
5. Garnish with herbs.

*8- or 9-inch pie plates

Makes: 3-4 servings (2-2½ cups)

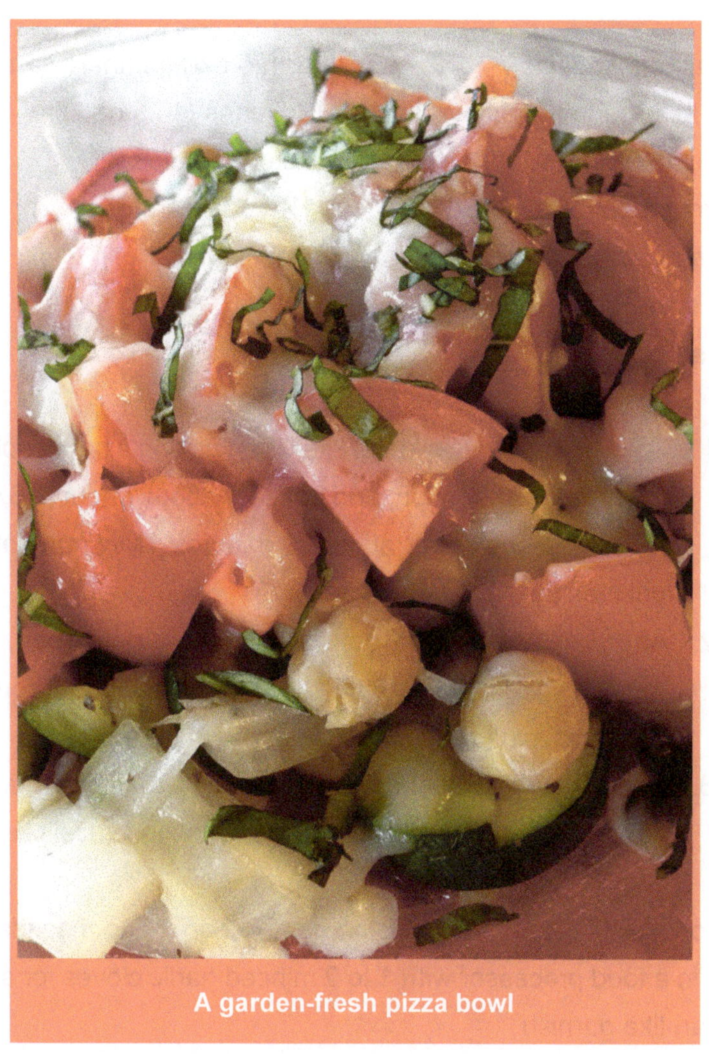

A garden-fresh pizza bowl

EASY SPAGHETTI

1 spaghetti squash
½-¾ lb. ground turkey breast (white/lean), browned
6-8 mushrooms, sliced and sautéed
½-¾ sweet onion, chopped and sautéed
1 jar (25 oz.) marinara sauce OR 2 cans (14.5 oz.) fire roasted tomatoes
1-1½ cups Parmesan cheese, grated*

1. Poke squash with a knife, like when baking a potato, place in shallow baking dish, and bake for about 1 hour at 375°F, rotating squash after about 30 minutes. Continue baking until tender.
2. After baking, slice off both ends, cut squash open, and remove seeds. With a fork, separate out spaghetti squash "noodles" and lightly butter or toss with olive oil.
3. Top with turkey, mushrooms, onions, fire roasted tomatoes or marinara sauce, and sprinkle with cheese. Delicious!

*Optional. For a dairy-free version, finely chop 1 cup macadamia nuts in a food processor with 1 to 2 minced garlic cloves for a parmesan-like garnish.

Makes: 6–8 servings (1½ cups)

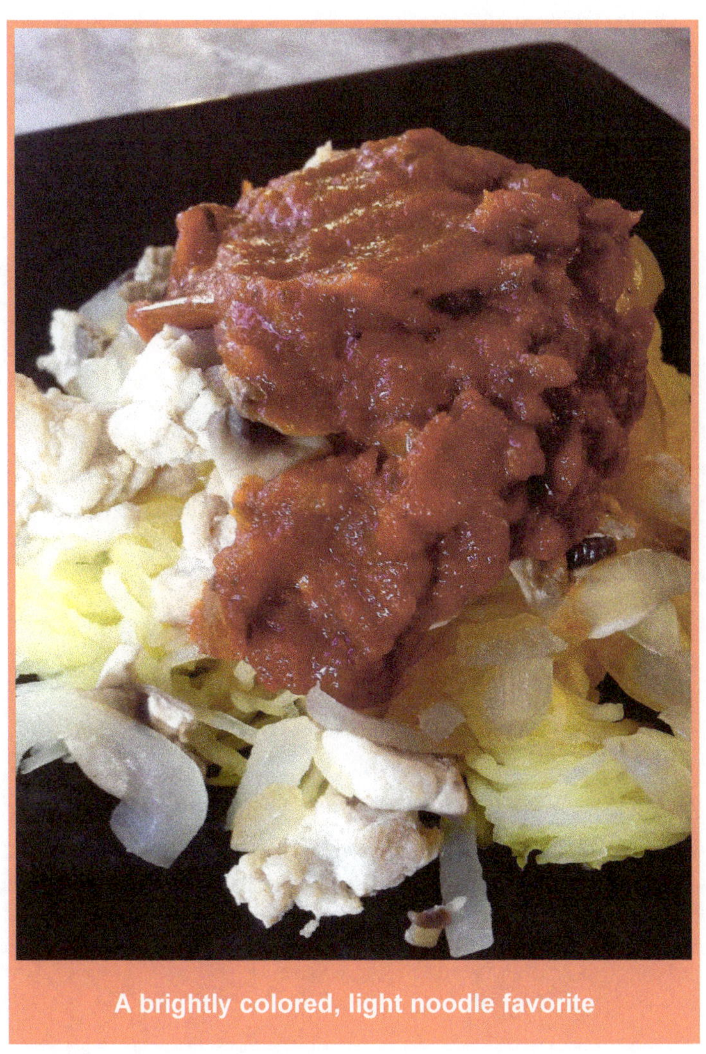

A brightly colored, light noodle favorite

FISH TACO WRAPS

1-1½ lbs. fresh or frozen white-fish fillets (wild cod, halibut, or other mild fish)
½ teaspoon garlic powder
½ teaspoon cumin
¼ teaspoon oregano
1 teaspoon chili powder
½ teaspoon onion powder
Cayenne and black pepper, to taste
½ teaspoon sea salt
1 head green cabbage*
½ onion, chopped
4-6 sweet mini peppers, sliced
¼-½ bunch fresh cilantro, chopped
1-2 avocados, sliced
Lime wedges

Creamy Taco Sauce

¼ cup sour cream or plain Greek yogurt**
1½ tablespoons lime juice
½ teaspoon raw honey
½ teaspoon fresh minced garlic
Cayenne and sea salt to taste

1. Combine spices in small bowl and sprinkle on both sides of the fish.
2. Bake or panfry until fillets flake with a fork.
3. While fish cooks, prep cabbage and Creamy Taco Sauce. Slice cabbage in half, rinse outer leaves, and carefully peel apart layers for "wraps."
4. Creamy Taco Sauce: in small bowl, combine all ingredients and stir until smooth.

5. Make tacos: fill cabbage leaves with fish, then layer onions, peppers, cilantro, and avocado. Drizzle with fresh lime juice or Creamy Taco Sauce. Roll or fold.
6. Also delicious served with black beans on the side or even added inside.

*Variation: Wrap with warm organic corn tortillas instead, using chopped cabbage inside.

**For dairy-free version, use smoothly mashed avocado thinned with water to desired consistency.

Makes: 4 servings

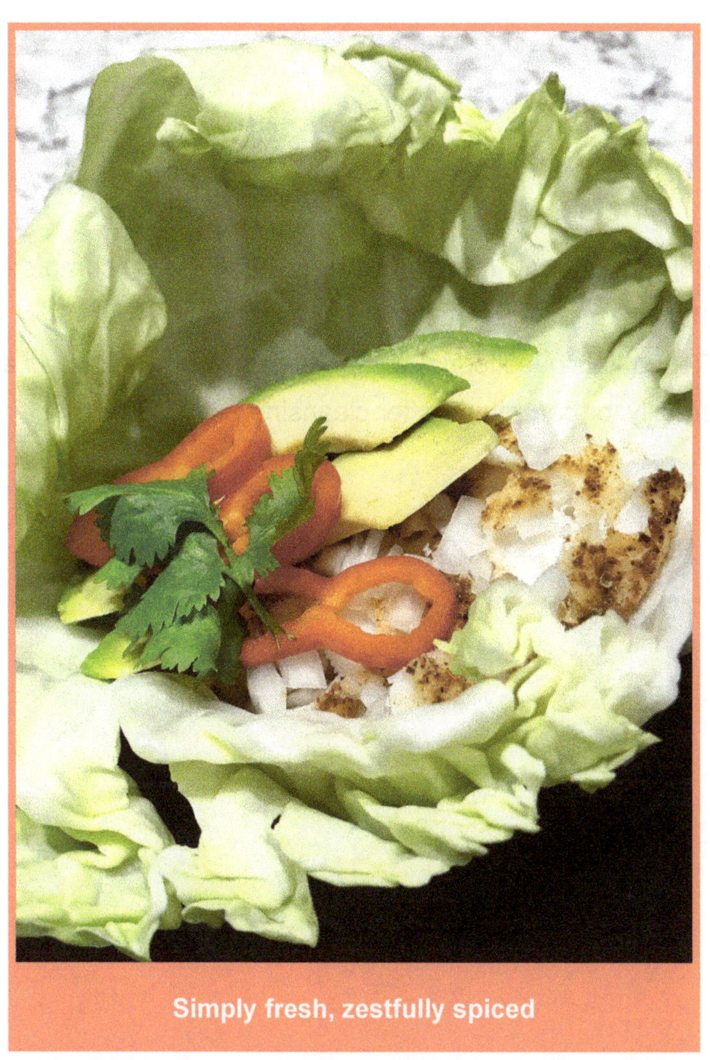

Simply fresh, zestfully spiced

Symptom Tracker

Before you start nutrition or lifestyle changes, complete the questionnaire to help track your progress.

Repeat this questionnaire after three to four weeks, and again seasonally, or before and after cleansing.

Scale: 0 (none) to 5 (severe/frequent)

	DATE:	DATE:	DATE:	DATE:
WEIGHT				
Binge eating/drinking	0 1 2 3 4 5	0 1 2 3 4 5	0 1 2 3 4 5	0 1 2 3 4 5
Excessive weight	0 1 2 3 4 5	0 1 2 3 4 5	0 1 2 3 4 5	0 1 2 3 4 5
Compulsive eating	0 1 2 3 4 5	0 1 2 3 4 5	0 1 2 3 4 5	0 1 2 3 4 5
Water retention	0 1 2 3 4 5	0 1 2 3 4 5	0 1 2 3 4 5	0 1 2 3 4 5
Underweight	0 1 2 3 4 5	0 1 2 3 4 5	0 1 2 3 4 5	0 1 2 3 4 5
TOTAL				
ENERGY/ACTIVITY				
Fatigue, sluggishness	0 1 2 3 4 5	0 1 2 3 4 5	0 1 2 3 4 5	0 1 2 3 4 5
Apathy, lethargy	0 1 2 3 4 5	0 1 2 3 4 5	0 1 2 3 4 5	0 1 2 3 4 5
Hyperactivity	0 1 2 3 4 5	0 1 2 3 4 5	0 1 2 3 4 5	0 1 2 3 4 5
Restlessness	0 1 2 3 4 5	0 1 2 3 4 5	0 1 2 3 4 5	0 1 2 3 4 5
Frequent illness	0 1 2 3 4 5	0 1 2 3 4 5	0 1 2 3 4 5	0 1 2 3 4 5
TOTAL				
EMOTIONS				
Mood swings	0 1 2 3 4 5	0 1 2 3 4 5	0 1 2 3 4 5	0 1 2 3 4 5
Anxiety, fear, nervousness	0 1 2 3 4 5	0 1 2 3 4 5	0 1 2 3 4 5	0 1 2 3 4 5
Anger, irritability	0 1 2 3 4 5	0 1 2 3 4 5	0 1 2 3 4 5	0 1 2 3 4 5
Depression	0 1 2 3 4 5	0 1 2 3 4 5	0 1 2 3 4 5	0 1 2 3 4 5
TOTAL				
MIND				
Poor memory	0 1 2 3 4 5	0 1 2 3 4 5	0 1 2 3 4 5	0 1 2 3 4 5
Poor concentration	0 1 2 3 4 5	0 1 2 3 4 5	0 1 2 3 4 5	0 1 2 3 4 5
Poor coordination	0 1 2 3 4 5	0 1 2 3 4 5	0 1 2 3 4 5	0 1 2 3 4 5
Difficulty making decisions	0 1 2 3 4 5	0 1 2 3 4 5	0 1 2 3 4 5	0 1 2 3 4 5
Learning disabilities	0 1 2 3 4 5	0 1 2 3 4 5	0 1 2 3 4 5	0 1 2 3 4 5
TOTAL				
DIGESTION				
Nausea or vomiting	0 1 2 3 4 5	0 1 2 3 4 5	0 1 2 3 4 5	0 1 2 3 4 5
Diarrhea	0 1 2 3 4 5	0 1 2 3 4 5	0 1 2 3 4 5	0 1 2 3 4 5
Constipation	0 1 2 3 4 5	0 1 2 3 4 5	0 1 2 3 4 5	0 1 2 3 4 5
Bloating	0 1 2 3 4 5	0 1 2 3 4 5	0 1 2 3 4 5	0 1 2 3 4 5
Belching, flatulence	0 1 2 3 4 5	0 1 2 3 4 5	0 1 2 3 4 5	0 1 2 3 4 5
Heartburn	0 1 2 3 4 5	0 1 2 3 4 5	0 1 2 3 4 5	0 1 2 3 4 5
TOTAL				
MOUTH/THROAT				
Chronic coughing	0 1 2 3 4 5	0 1 2 3 4 5	0 1 2 3 4 5	0 1 2 3 4 5
Throat congestion	0 1 2 3 4 5	0 1 2 3 4 5	0 1 2 3 4 5	0 1 2 3 4 5
Sore throat, hoarseness	0 1 2 3 4 5	0 1 2 3 4 5	0 1 2 3 4 5	0 1 2 3 4 5
Canker sores	0 1 2 3 4 5	0 1 2 3 4 5	0 1 2 3 4 5	0 1 2 3 4 5
TOTAL				

Skin				
Acne	0 1 2 3 4 5	0 1 2 3 4 5	0 1 2 3 4 5	0 1 2 3 4 5
Hives, rashes, dry skin	0 1 2 3 4 5	0 1 2 3 4 5	0 1 2 3 4 5	0 1 2 3 4 5
Hair loss	0 1 2 3 4 5	0 1 2 3 4 5	0 1 2 3 4 5	0 1 2 3 4 5
Flushing or hot flashes	0 1 2 3 4 5	0 1 2 3 4 5	0 1 2 3 4 5	0 1 2 3 4 5
Excessive sweating	0 1 2 3 4 5	0 1 2 3 4 5	0 1 2 3 4 5	0 1 2 3 4 5
TOTAL				
Joints/Muscles				
Pain or aches in joints	0 1 2 3 4 5	0 1 2 3 4 5	0 1 2 3 4 5	0 1 2 3 4 5
Arthritis	0 1 2 3 4 5	0 1 2 3 4 5	0 1 2 3 4 5	0 1 2 3 4 5
Stiffness, limited movement	0 1 2 3 4 5	0 1 2 3 4 5	0 1 2 3 4 5	0 1 2 3 4 5
Pain, aches in muscles	0 1 2 3 4 5	0 1 2 3 4 5	0 1 2 3 4 5	0 1 2 3 4 5
Feeling weak/tired	0 1 2 3 4 5	0 1 2 3 4 5	0 1 2 3 4 5	0 1 2 3 4 5
TOTAL				
Head				
Headaches	0 1 2 3 4 5	0 1 2 3 4 5	0 1 2 3 4 5	0 1 2 3 4 5
Faintness	0 1 2 3 4 5	0 1 2 3 4 5	0 1 2 3 4 5	0 1 2 3 4 5
Dizziness	0 1 2 3 4 5	0 1 2 3 4 5	0 1 2 3 4 5	0 1 2 3 4 5
Insomnia	0 1 2 3 4 5	0 1 2 3 4 5	0 1 2 3 4 5	0 1 2 3 4 5
TOTAL				
Heart				
Skipped heartbeats	0 1 2 3 4 5	0 1 2 3 4 5	0 1 2 3 4 5	0 1 2 3 4 5
Rabid heartbeats	0 1 2 3 4 5	0 1 2 3 4 5	0 1 2 3 4 5	0 1 2 3 4 5
Chest pain	0 1 2 3 4 5	0 1 2 3 4 5	0 1 2 3 4 5	0 1 2 3 4 5
TOTAL				
Nose				
Stuffy nose	0 1 2 3 4 5	0 1 2 3 4 5	0 1 2 3 4 5	0 1 2 3 4 5
Sinus problems	0 1 2 3 4 5	0 1 2 3 4 5	0 1 2 3 4 5	0 1 2 3 4 5
Hay fever	0 1 2 3 4 5	0 1 2 3 4 5	0 1 2 3 4 5	0 1 2 3 4 5
TOTAL				
Eyes				
Watery, itchy eyes	0 1 2 3 4 5	0 1 2 3 4 5	0 1 2 3 4 5	0 1 2 3 4 5
Swollen, puffy eyes	0 1 2 3 4 5	0 1 2 3 4 5	0 1 2 3 4 5	0 1 2 3 4 5
Dark circles under eyes	0 1 2 3 4 5	0 1 2 3 4 5	0 1 2 3 4 5	0 1 2 3 4 5
TOTAL				
Ears				
Itchy ears	0 1 2 3 4 5	0 1 2 3 4 5	0 1 2 3 4 5	0 1 2 3 4 5
Earaches, ear infections	0 1 2 3 4 5	0 1 2 3 4 5	0 1 2 3 4 5	0 1 2 3 4 5
Drainage from ears	0 1 2 3 4 5	0 1 2 3 4 5	0 1 2 3 4 5	0 1 2 3 4 5
Ringing in ears, hearing loss	0 1 2 3 4 5	0 1 2 3 4 5	0 1 2 3 4 5	0 1 2 3 4 5
TOTAL				
Lungs				
Chest congestion	0 1 2 3 4 5	0 1 2 3 4 5	0 1 2 3 4 5	0 1 2 3 4 5
Asthma, bronchitis	0 1 2 3 4 5	0 1 2 3 4 5	0 1 2 3 4 5	0 1 2 3 4 5
Difficulty breathing	0 1 2 3 4 5	0 1 2 3 4 5	0 1 2 3 4 5	0 1 2 3 4 5
TOTAL				
GRAND TOTAL				

Lifestyle Log

1. Circle the **Day** of the week and fill in the **Date** you are recording.
2. Include the **Time** you eat or drink.
3. Record everything you eat and drink, listing each **Food/ Beverage** item individually. For example, if you are eating a salad, list everything that is on the salad (e.g., romaine lettuce, tomato, cucumber, croutons, sunflower seeds, salad dressing). If the food comes from a can, package, or restaurant, include the brand name. Be as specific as possible.
4. Record the **Amount** of the food/beverage you eat. Use measuring cups and spoons or scales for accuracy. Portion sizes may surprise you.
5. Add **Exercise Type and Length**.
6. Include **Total Water Intake** (measured in cups, quarts, or ounces).
7. Record daily form(s) of **Relaxation** (e.g., music therapy, quality time with friends, prayer, art, hobbies).
8. Note **Hours of Sleep** and any comments on **Sleep Quality**.

Record relevant information as often as needed to find patterns, track progress, and stay accountable.

	S M T W Th F S		Date: ___________
Time	**Food/Beverage**	**Amount**	**Exercise** **Type and Length**
			Total Water Intake
			Relaxation
			Hours and Quality of Sleep

Mindful Eating Journal

Journal your hunger levels and the emotions* you experience around the times you eat. At the end of the day, review and summarize the emotions of the day. Then, take a few minutes to process, reflect on, and settle the events, triggers, and happenings of the day.

Day:		
Meal/Time	**Hunger** 0 – 5 starving	**Emotions***

Daily Emotions Summary

*stressed, tired, happy, lonely, bored, angry, anxious, ignored, depressed, sad, afraid, confused, overwhelmed, embarrassed, shy, left out, hysterical, exhausted, guilty, frustrated, rejected, jealous, ashamed, worried, hopeful, irritable, numb

Journal

About the Author

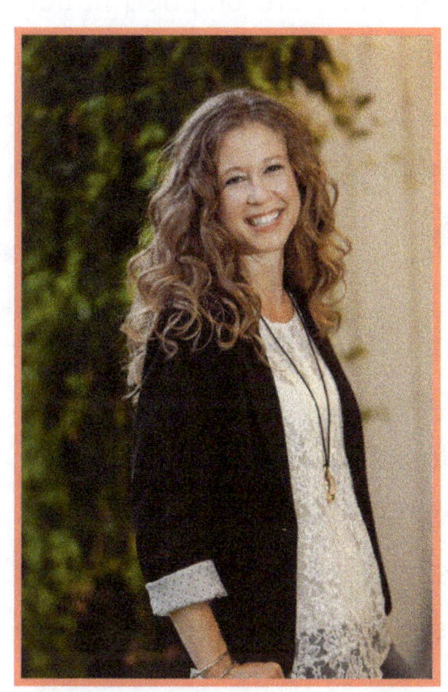

Alisha Chasey began her college education at Virginia Tech, earned her nutrition degrees at the University of Arizona (BS) and Arizona State University (MS), and holds credentials as a registered dietitian, certified nutrition specialist, and associate raw foods chef. Her professional clinical experience with dialysis, a comprehensive cancer-care clinic, and her own persistent health issues (chronic fatigue, food allergies and indigestion, cystic acne) taught her the real-life impact of nutrition and lifestyle on peoples' short and long-term health. On her own journey, she explored traditional, alternative, and complementary medicine, and also experimented with every kind of "-free" diet, vegan and raw foods, juicing, cleansing, and more. As a self-proclaimed "dessert queen," she quickly felt deprived and dissatisfied as she faced the epic task of transforming her "sweet-tooth" eating. She soon discovered through her journey in the kitchen that true health and wholeness come from making choices on every level—physical, emotional, and spiritual.

Innocent Indulgence® was birthed out of Alisha's passion to help others experience radiant, healthy living, to live out their destinies, and to love their lives, while eating with "all of the yum and none of the guilt" every step of the way. She loves using desserts to promote the deliciousness of balanced, plant-rich eating. For a season, Innocent Indulgence's desserts were shipped nationwide and available at Arizona's Whole Foods Markets®, New Frontiers®, and local restaurants. Now you can make some of them in your own kitchen. Living healthy and feeling good has never been sweeter or more satisfying. You really can indulge innocently!

Alisha now enjoys clear skin and lots of energy, eating balanced and clean, and being free from food allergies. She loves being outdoors, snapping flower photos, dabbling with watercolors, sipping coffee, and spending time with family and friends. She's focused on sharing the secrets she's learned about wellness and healing in one-on-one and group sessions, so *you* can make healthy daily, doable, and delicious.

If you want to experience and learn more about this life-changing key to radiant living, visit InnocentIndulgence.com/secret.

Have you been encouraged, found hope, or experienced healing through this reading? I'd love to hear your story. You can contact me at info@InnocentIndulgence.com or through my website InnocentIndulgence.com.

Visit InnocentIndulgence.com for additional tips, recipes, and secrets.

Let's stay connected:
Facebook: Innocent Indulgence
Twitter: @InnocentIndulge
Instagram: innocentindulgence

Coming soon—a sequel with more steps to radiant living!

Watch for *ResparkleU*, an online body reset course – Coming Spring 2018

Endnotes

1 "Chronic Disease Overview," Centers for Disease Control and Prevention, last modified August 26, 2015. http://www.cdc.gov/chronicdisease/overview/index.htm#ref1.

2 Brian W. Ward, Jeannine S. Schiller, and Richard A. Goodman, "Multiple Chronic Conditions Among US Adults: A 2012 update," *Preventing Chronic Disease* 11 (2014), doi: 10.5888/pcd11.130389.

3 Cheryl D. Fryar, Te-Ching Chen, and Xianfen Li, "Prevalence of Uncontrolled Risk Factors for Cardiovascular Disease: United States, 1999–2010," NCHS Data Brief, no. 103 (2012), https://www.cdc.gov/nchs/products/databriefs/db103.htm.

4 "Chronic Disease Overview," Center for Disease Control, last modified August 26, 2015. http://www.cdc.gov/chronicdisease/overview/index.htm#ref1.

5 "Adult Obesity Facts," Centers for Disease Control and Prevention, last modified September 21, 2015, http://www.cdc.gov/obesity/data/adult.html.

6 "Obesity and Overweight," Centers for Disease Control and Prevention, last modified September 30, 2015, http://www.cdc.gov/nchs/fastats/obesity-overweight.htm.

7 Y Clair Wang et al., "Health and Economic Burden of the Projected Obesity Trends in the USA and the UK," *The Lancet* 378, no. 9793 (2011): 815–825, doi: 10.1016/S0140-6736(11)60814-3.

8 "Division of Nutrition, Physical Activity, and Obesity—Childhood Obesity Facts," Centers for Disease Control and Prevention, last modified June 19, 2015, http://www.cdc.gov/obesity/data/childhood.html.

9 Eric A. Finkelstein et al., "Annual Medical Spending Attributable to Obesity: Payer-and Service-Specific Estimates," *Health Affairs* 28 (2009): w822–w831, accessed December 23, 2013 http://content.healthaffairs.org/content/28/5/w822.full.html.

10 *2010 Shape of the Nation Report*, National Association for Sport and Physical Education, accessed July 2016, http://www.shapeamerica.org/advocacy/son/upload/Shape-of-the-Nation-2010-Final.pdf.

11 "The Healthcare Costs of Obesity," *the State of Obesity*, accessed June 2017, http://stateofobesity.org/healthcare-costs-obesity/.

12 Kate Kelland, "A Third of People Worldwide Are Either Undernourished or Overweight," *Business Insider*, June 14, 2016, http://www.businessinsider.com/r-too-fat-too-thin-report-finds-malnutrition-fuels-disease-worldwide-2016-6.

13 "Diabetes in the United States," Centers for Disease Control and Prevention, last modified 2014, http://www.cdc.gov/diabetes/pubs/images/diabetes-infographic.jpg.

14 "National Diabetes Statistics Report: Estimates of Diabetes and Its Burden in the United States," Division of Diabetes Translation, Centers for Disease Control and Prevention (2014), https://www.cdc.gov/diabetes/pubs/statsreport14/national-diabetes-report-web.pdf.

15 "Statistics About Diabetes," American Diabetes Association, *National Diabetes Statistics Report*, released June 10, 2014, http://www.diabetes.org/diabetes-basics/statistics/.

16 "Nerve Damage (Diabetic Neuropathies)," The National Institute of Diabetes and Digestive and Kidney Diseases, accessed January 13, 2016, http://diabetes.niddk.nih.gov/dm/pubs/neuropathies/.

17 "Diabetes in the United States," Centers for Disease Control and Prevention, last modified 2014, http://www.cdc.gov/diabetes/pubs/images/diabetes-infographic.jpg.

18 "National Diabetes Statistics Report: Estimates of Diabetes and Its Burden in the United States," Division of Diabetes Translation, Centers for Disease Control and Prevention (2014), https://www.cdc.gov/diabetes/pubs/statsreport14/national-diabetes-report-web.pdf.

19 "Food Allergy Facts and Statistics for the U.S.," Food Allergy Research and Education, accessed 2015, http://www.foodallergy.org/document.doc?id=194.

20 "Facts and Statistics," Food Allergy Research and Education, accessed 2015, http://www.foodallergy.org/facts-and-stats.

21 Kristin D. Jackson, LaJeana D. Howie, and Lara J. Akinbami, "Trends in Allergic Conditions Among Children: United States, 1997–2011," NCHS Data Brief, no. 121 (2013), https://www.cdc.gov/nchs/products/databriefs/db121.htm.

22 Amy M. Branum and Susan L. Lukacs, "Food Allergy Among U.S. Children: Trends in Prevalence and Hospitalizations," NCHS Data Brief, no. 10 (2008), http://www.cdc.gov/nchs/data/databriefs/db10.htm.

23 "Facts and Statistics," Food Allergy Research and Education, accessed 2015, http://www.foodallergy.org/facts-and-stats.

24 Ruchi Gupta et al, "The High Economic Burden of Childhood Food Allergy in the United States." *The Journal of Allergy and Clinical Immunology* 109, no. 2 (2012): A1–A162, doi: 10.1016/j.jaci.2012.12.1464.

25 "Celiac Disease: Fast Facts," Beyond Celiac, accessed January 13, 2016, http://www.celiaccentral.org/celiac-disease/facts-and-figures/.

26 "Celiac Disease Facts and Figures," University of Chicago Celiac Disease Center, accessed January 13, 2016, http://www.uchospitals.edu/pdf/uch_007937.pdf.

27 "Gluten-Free Market Trends," The Gluten Free Agency, accessed January 13, 2016, http://thegluten-freeagency.com/gluten-free-market-trends/.

28 Jon Baio, "Prevalence of Autism Spectrum Disorder Among Children Aged 8 Years—Autism and Developmental Disabilities Monitoring Network, 11 Sites, United States, 2010." *Surveillance Summaries: Morbidity and Mortality Weekly Report* 63, no. SS02 (March 28, 2014): 1–21, http://www.cdc.gov/mmwr/preview/mmwrhtml/ss6302a1.htm?s_cid=ss6302a1_w.

29 Karen Weintraub, "Autism Rates Soar, Now Affects 1 in 68 Children," *USA Today*, March 27, 2014, http://www.usatoday.com/story/news/nation/2014/03/27/autism-rates-rise/6957815/.

30 Barbara Starfield, "Is US Health Really the Best in the World?" *Journal of the American Medical Association* 284, no. 4 (2000): 483–485, doi: 10.1001/jama.284.4.483.

31 Bruce Horovitz and Julie Appleby, "Prescription Drug Costs are Up; So are TV Ads Promoting Them," *USA Today,* March 16, 2017, https://www.usatoday.com/story/money/2017/03/16/prescription-drug-costs-up-tv-ads/99203878/.

32 John Henning Schumann, "Those TV Drug Ads Distract Us from the Medical Care We Need," *NPR,* April 29, 2017, http://www.npr.org/sections/health-shots/2017/04/29/525877472/those-tv-drug-ads-distract-us-from-the-medical-care-we-need.

33 "Exercise or Physical Activity," Centers for Disease Control and Prevention, last modified July 20, 2015, http://www.cdc.gov/nchs/fastats/exercise.htm.

34 "Facts and Statistics," President's Council on Fitness, Sports & Nutrition, accessed 2015, http://www.fitness.gov/resource-center/facts-and-statistics/#footnote-12.

35 "Healthy People 2010," Centers for Disease Control and Prevention, last modified October 14, 2009, http://www.cdc.gov/nchs/healthy_people/hp2010.htm.

36 National Association for Sport and Physical Education, *The Fitness Equation: Physical Activity + Balanced Diet = Fit Kids* (Reston, VA: National Association for Sport and Physical Education, 1999).

37 Victoria J. Rideout, Ulla G. Foehr, and Donald F. Roberts, "Generation M2: Media in the Lives of 8- to 18-Year-Olds," A Kaiser Family Foundation Study (2010), http://files.eric.ed.gov/fulltext/ED527859.pdf.

38 "Where's the Sodium?" *CDC Vital Signs*, last modified 2012, http://www.cdc.gov/VitalSigns/pdf/2012-02-vitalsigns.pdf.

39 "Adults Meeting Fruit and Vegetable Intake Recommendations—United States, 2013," *Morbidity and Mortality Weekly Reports*, 64, no. 26 (July 10, 2015): 709–713, http://www.cdc.gov/mmwr/preview/mmwrhtml/mm6426a1.htm.

40 Maggie Fox, "You're Still Not Eating Enough Vegetables," NBC News, July 9, 2015, http://www.nbcnews.com/health/diet-fitness/youre-still-not-eating-enough-vegetables-n389466.

41 "Usual Dietary Intakes: Food Intakes, U.S. Population, 2007–10," National Cancer Institute, Division of Cancer Control & Population Sciences, last modified May 20, 2015, http://appliedresearch.cancer.gov/diet/usualintakes/pop/2007-10.

42 "One Sweet Nation," *U.S. News & World Report*, October 15, 2008, http://health.usnews.com/usnews/health/articles/050328/28sugar.b_print.htm.

43 Alice G. Walton, "How Much Sugar Are Americans Eating?" *Forbes,* August 30, 2012, http://www.forbes.com/sites/alicegwalton/2012/08/30/how-much-sugar-are-americans-eating-infographic/#26af7a9f1f71.

44 Biing-Hwan Lin, Jean C. Buzby, Tobenna D. Anekwe, and Jeanine T. Bentley, "U.S. Food Commodity Consumption Broken Down by Demographics, 1994-2008," USDA Economic Research Service, Economic Research Report, no. 206 (March 2016), https://www.ers.usda.gov/webdocs/publications/err206/57057_err-206.pdf?v=42459.

45 "Food Availability and Consumption," USDA Economic Research Service, last modified October 18, 2017, https://www.ers.usda.gov/data-products/ag-and-food-statistics-charting-the-essentials/food-availability-and-consumption.

46 Beth Hoffman, "One Way to Be Healthier: Don't Eat Like the Average American" *Forbes*, March 18, 2013, https://www.forbes.com/sites/bethhoffman/2013/03/18/one-way-to-be-healthier-dont-eat-like-the-average-american/#b7cd2d32bd6e.

47 Tulip Mazumda, "Obesity Boom 'Fueling Rise in Malnutrition.'" BBC News, June 14, 2016, http://www.bbc.com/news/health-36518770.

48 Caroline Leaf, *Think and Eat Yourself Smart: A Neuroscientific Approach to a Sharper Mind and Healthier Life*, (Grand Rapids, MI: Baker Books, 2016), 144–153.

49 M. Katherine Hoy, EdD, RD and Joseph D. Goldman, MA, "Fiber Intake of the US Population - What We Eat in America, NHANES 2009-2010," Food Surveys Research Group Dietary Data Brief, no. 12 (Sept 2014), https://www.ars.usda.gov/ARSUserFiles/80400530/pdf/dbrief/12_fiber_intake_0910.pdf.

50 "2010 Dietary Guidelines for Americans," United States Department of Agriculture, accessed 2015, http://www.cnpp.usda.gov/DietaryGuidelines.

51 "Canada's Food Guide," Health Canada, last modified February 5, 2007, http://www.hc-sc.gc.ca/fn-an/food-guide-aliment/basics-base/quantit-eng.php.

52 Physicians Committee for Responsible Medicine, accessed 2015, http://www.pcrm.org/health/veginfo/vsk/food_groups.html.

53 James McCormack, "How Many Servings of Fruits and Vegetables Should We Eat a Day?" *HuffPost Living*, October 31, 2014, http://www.huffingtonpost.ca/james-mccormack/fruits-and-vegetables_b_6071310.html.

54 "The Nutrition Source—Vegetables and Fruits," Harvard T.H. Chan School of Public Health, accessed January 14, 2016 http://www.hsph.harvard.edu/nutritionsource/what-should-you-eat/vegetables-and-fruits/.

55 Rui Hai Lui, "Health Benefits of Fruit and Vegetables Are from Additive and Synergistic Combinations of Phytochemicals," *American Journal of Clinical Nutrition* 78, no. 3 (2003): 517S–520S, http://ajcn.nutrition.org/content/78/3/517S.abstract.

56 Pivonka E. Van Duyn, "Overview of the Health Benefits of Fruit and Vegetable Consumption for the Dietetics Professional: Selected Literature," *Journal of the American Dietetic Association* 100, no.12 (2000): 1,511–21, https://www.ncbi.nlm.nih.gov/pubmed/11138444.

57 "UCL Study Finds New Evidence Linking Fruit and Vegetable Consumption with Lower Mortality," University College London, April 1 2014. http://www.ucl.ac.uk/news/news-articles/0414/010413-fruit-veg-consumption-death-risk.

58 Oyinlola Oyebode et al., "Fruit and Vegetable Consumption and All-Cause, Cancer and CVD Mortality: Analysis of Health Survey for England Data," *Journal of Epidemiology & Community Health* 68, no. 9 (2014): 856–862, http://jech.bmj.com/content/68/9/856.

59 Michael Downey, "Olive Oil: Powerful Protection Against Aging and Mortality," *Life Extensions Magazine*, August 2014, http://www.lifeextension.com/magazine/2014/8/olive-oil-powerful-protection-against-aging-and-mortality/page-01.

60 "Olive Oil, Extra Virgin" World's Healthiest Foods, accessed 2017, http://www.whfoods.com/genpage.php?tname=foodspice&dbid=132.

61 "Types of Fats," The Nutrition Source, Harvard T.H. Chan School of Public Health, accessed 2017, https://www.hsph.harvard.edu/nutritionsource/types-of-fat/.

62 James J. DiNicolantonio, Sean C. Lucan, and James H. O'Keefe, "The Evidence for Saturated Fat and for Sugar Related to Coronary

Heart Disease," *Progress in Cardiovascular Diseases* 58, no. 5 (2015): 464–472, doi: 10.1016/j.pcad.2015.11.006. https://www.sciencedaily.com/releases/2016/01/160113103318.htm.

63 Anahad O'Connor, "How the Sugar Industry Shifted Blame to Fat," *The New York Times,* September 12, 2016, http://www.nytimes.com/2016/09/13/well/eat/how-the-sugar-industry-shifted-blame-to-fat.html?_r=0.

64 "Talking About Trans Fat: What You Need to Know," U.S. Food and Drug Administration, last updated May 22, 2016, http://www.fda.gov/Food/ResourcesForYou/Consumers/ucm079609.htm.

65 J. H. Kelly Jr., J. Sabate, "Nuts and Coronary Heart Disease: An Epidemiological Perspective," *British Journal of Nutrition* 99, no. 2 (2008): 447–448. PMID:17125535.

66 Laura A. Yochum, Aaron R. Folsom, and Lawrence H. Kushi, "Intake of Antioxidant Vitamins and Risk of Death from Stroke in Postmenopausal Women," *The American Journal of Clinical Nutrition* 72, no. 2 (2000): 476–483, http://ajcn.nutrition.org/content/72/2/476.full.

67 R Jiang et al., "Nut and Peanut Butter Consumption and Risk of Type 2 Diabetes in Women," *Journal of the American Medical Association* 288, no. 20 (2002): 2,554–2,560, PMID: 12444862.

68 S. M. Zhang et al., "Intakes of Vitamins E and C, Carotenoids, Vitamin Supplements, and PD Risk," *Neurology* 59, no. 8 (2002): 1,161–1,169, doi: 10.1212/01.WNL.0000028688.75881.12.

69 J. M. Seddon, J. Cote, and B. Rosner, "Progression of Age-Related Macular Degeneration: Association with Dietary Fat, Transunsaturated Fat, Nuts, and Fish Intake," *The Archives of Ophthalmology* 121, no. 12 (2003): 1,728–1,737, doi: 10.1001/archopht.121.12.1728.

70 Chung-Jyi Tsai et al., "Frequent Nut Consumption and Decreased Risk of Cholecystectomy in Women," *The American Journal of Clinical Nutrition* 80, no. 1 (2004): 76–81, http://ajcn.nutrition.org/content/80/1/76.full.

71 M. Bes-Rastrollo et al., "Nut Consumption and Weight Gain in a Mediterranean Cohort: The SUN Study," *Obesity* 15, no. 1 (2007): 107–116, PMID: 17228038.

72 Christine M. Kaefer and John A. Milner, "Herbs and Spices in Cancer Prevention and Treatment," in *Herbal Medicine: Biomolecular and Clinical Aspects*, 2nd ed., ed. Iris F. F. Benzie and Sissi Wachtel-Galor (Boca Raton, FL: CRC Press, 2010) accessed January 14, 2016, http://www.ncbi.nlm.nih.gov/books/NBK92774/.

73 "Turmeric," World's Healthiest Foods, accessed 2015, http://www.whfoods.com/genpage.php?tname=foodspice&dbid=78.

74 "Inflammation (Chronic)," LifeExtension, http://www.lifeextension.com/Protocols/Health-Concerns/Chronic-Inflammation/Page-02.

75 Nancy Appleton and G. N. Jacobs, "141 Reasons Sugar Ruins Your Health," Nancy Appleton Books, last updated 2015, https://nancyappleton.com/141-reasons-sugar-ruins-your-health/.

76 G Vighi, et al., "Allergy and the gastrointestinal system," *Clin Exp Immunol.* 2008 Sep; 153(Suppl 1): 3–6. doi: 10.1111/j.1365-2249.2008.03713.x. https://www.ncbi.nlm.nih.gov/pmc/articles/PMC2515351/.

77 David Perlmutter, "Elevated Blood Sugar Shrinks the Brain," accessed September 2016, http://www.drperlmutter.com/elevated-blood-sugar-shrinks-brain/.

78 Lucia Kerti, et al, "Higher Glucose Levels Associated with Lower Memory and Reduced Hippocampal Microstructure," *Journal of Neurology* 81, no. 20 (2013): 1,746–1,752, doi: 10.1212/01.wnl.0000435561.00234.ee.

79 "Diabetes and Dementia—Is There a Connection?" Alzheimer Society Canada, accessed February 2016, http://www.alzheimer.ca/en/About-dementia/Alzheimer-s-disease/Risk-factors/Diabetes-dementia-connection.

80 Wendy Brundige and Eric Noll, "The Science of Food Cravings," ABC News, November 14, 2009, http://abcnews.go.com/GMA/Weekend/junk-food-addictive-illegal-drugs/story?id=9083548.

81 Jennifer A. Nettleton, et al., "Diet Soda Intake and Risk of Incident Metabolic Syndrome and Type 2 Diabetes in the Multi-Ethnic Study of Atherosclerosis (MESA)," Diabetes Care 2009 Apr; 32(4): 688-694, doi.org/10.2337/dc08-1799. Accessed 2017, *American Diabetes Association,* http://care.diabetesjournals.org/content/32/4/688.

82 Mark Hyman, "How Diet Soda Makes You Fat (and Other Food and Diet Industry Secrets)," *The Huffington Post*, March

7, 2013, http://www.huffingtonpost.com/dr-mark-hyman/diet-soda-health_b_2698494.html.

83 Guy Fagherazzi et al., "Consumption of Artificially and Sugar-Sweetened Beverages and Incident Type 2 Diabetes in European Prospective Investigation into Cancer and Nutrition Cohort," *The American Journal of Clinical Nutrition* 97, no. 3 (2013): 517–523, doi: 10.3945/ajcn.112.050997.

84 Richard D. Mattes and Barry M. Popkin, "Nonnutritive Sweetener Consumption in Humans: Effects on Appetite and Food Intake and Their Putative Mechanisms," *The American Journal of Clinical Nutrition* 89, no. 1 (2009): 1–14, doi: 10.3945/ajcn.2008.26792.

85 Mark Hyman, MD, "Why You Should Ditch Artificial Sweeteners," December 2, 2015, http://drhyman.com/blog/2015/12/02/why-you-should-ditch-artificial-sweeteners/.

86 "Artificial Sweeteners," Harvard T.H. Chan School of Public Health, *The Nutrition* Source, https://www.hsph.harvard.edu/nutritionsource/healthy-drinks/artificial-sweeteners/.

87 Jotham Suez et al., "Artificial Sweeteners Induce Glucose Intolerance by Altering the Gut Microbiota," *Nature* 514, no. 7521 (2014): 181–186, doi: 10.1038/nature13793.

88 Sharon P. G. Fowler, Ken Williams, and Helen P. Hazuda, "Diet Soda Intake Is Associated with Long-Term Increases in Waist Circumference in a Biethnic Cohort of Older Adults: The San Antonio Longitudinal Study of Aging," *Journal of the American Geriatrics Society* 63, no. 4 (2015): 708–715, doi: 10.1111/jgs.13376.

89 "Aspartame Studies," Mercola, http://aspartame.mercola.com/sites/aspartame/studies.aspx.

90 Derek Schramm, et al., "Honey with High Levels of Antioxidants Can Provide Protection to Healthy Human Subjects," *J. Agric. Food Chem.*, 2003, 51 (6), pp 1732–1735, doi: 10.1021/jf025928k http://pubs.acs.org/doi/abs/10.1021/jf025928k.

91 Jane Higdon, Ph.D., "Glycemic Index and Glycemic Load," *Linus Pauling Institute*, Oregon State University, last updated March 2016, http://lpi.oregonstate.edu/mic/food-beverages/glycemic-index-glycemic-load.

92 "Maple Syrup Nutrition," *Federation of Quebec Maple Syrup Producers*, last accessed, September 2017, http://www.purecanadamaple.com/benefits-of-maple-syrup/maple-syrup-nutrition/.

93 "Antioxidants in Maple Syrup," *Federation of Quebec Maple Syrup Producers*, last accessed, September 2017, http://www.purecanadamaple.com/benefits-of-maple-syrup/antioxidants-in-maple-syrup/.

94 "Celiac Disease Facts and Figures," The University of Chicago Medicine Celiac Disease Center, accessed June 2017, https://www.cureceliacdisease.org/wp-content/uploads/341_CDCFactSheets8_FactsFigures.pdf.

95 William Davis, *Wheat Belly: Lose the Wheat, Lose the Weight, and Find Your Path Back to Health* (New York: Rodale, 2011), 18-22.

96 Ibid., 34.

97 Ibid., 63.

98 William Davis, "The Gliadin Effect" January 14, 2012, http://www.wheatbellyblog.com/2012/01/the-gliadin-effect/comment-page-1.

99 Davis, *Wheat Belly: Lose the Wheat, Lose the Weight, and Find your Path Back to Health,* 50.

100 Leaf, *Think and Eat Yourself Smart*, 202–203.

101 Davis, *Wheat Belly, 43-187*.

102 "Food Allergies: What you Need to Know," US Food & Drug Administration, last updated April 5, 2017, https://www.fda.gov/food/resourcesforyou/consumers/ucm079311.htm.

103 "Scientific Report of the 2015 Dietary Guidelines Advisory Committee: Part D. Chapter 5: Food Sustainability and Safety – Continued," *Office of Disease Prevention and Health Promotion*, last updated May 2017, https://health.gov/dietaryguidelines/2015-scientific-report/10-chapter-5/d5-4.asp.

104 Stephanie Watson, "Tea: Drink to Your Health?" *Harvard Health Publications*, December 18, 2013, http://www.health.harvard.edu/blog/tea-drink-to-your-health-201312186947.

105 "Health Benefits Linked to Drinking Tea," *Harvard Health Publications*, September 2014, http://www.health.harvard.edu/press_releases/health-benefits-linked-to-drinking-tea.

106 Megan Ware, "Green Tea: Health Benefits, Side Effects, and Research," *Medical News Today*, last updated March 28, 2017, http://www.medicalnewstoday.com/articles/269538.php.

107 Leaf, *Think and Eat Yourself Smart*, 97.

108 "Stress Management for the Health of It," National Agricultural Safety Database, Clemson University Cooperative Extension Service, accessed February 2016, http://nasdonline.org/1445/d001245/stress-management-for-the-health-of-it.html.

109 Paul J. Rosch, "Job Stress: America's Leading Adult Health Problem," *USA Magazine*, May 1991.

110 Last accessed December 2015 http://www.cdc.gov/nasd/docs/d001201-d001300/d001245/d001245.html.

111 "America's #1 Health Problem," *The American Institute of Stress*, last accessed February 2017, https://www.stress.org/americas-1-health-problem/.

112 Don Colbert, MD, *Deadly Emotions* (Nashville: Thomas Nelson, 2003), 13.

113 "Stress and Eating," *American Psychological Association*, last accessed May 2017, http://www.apa.org/news/press/releases/stress/2013/eating.aspx.

114 Leaf, *Think and Eat Yourself Smart*, 84.

115 Ibid., 121.

116 Ibid., 123.

CPSIA information can be obtained
at www.ICGtesting.com
Printed in the USA
LVHW02s1234170118
562756LV00002BA/2/P